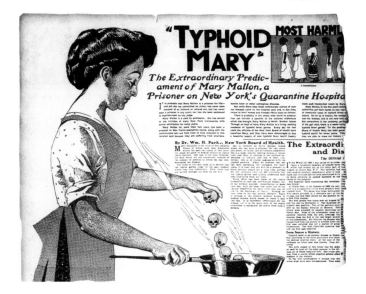

T Y P H O I D

The past, present and future of an ancient disease

CLAAS KIRCHHELLE

Für Emil

This edition © Scala Arts &
Heritage Publishers Ltd, 2022
Text © Oxford Vaccine Group, 2022

First published in 2022 by
Scala Arts & Heritage Publishers Ltd
305 Access House
141–157 Acre Lane
London SW2 5UA
www.scalapublishers.com

In association with
Oxford Vaccine Group
University of Oxford
Oxford OX3 7LE
www.ovg.ox.ac.uk

ISBN 978-1-78551-383-1

Edited by Neil Burkey
Designed by Andrew Barron
Printed and bound in Turkey

10 9 8 7 6 5 4 3 2 1

FRONTISPIECE
Mary Mallon, known as 'Typhoid Mary';
see page 53

Contents

CHAPTER ONE

Introduction: Fred Vincy's rash

I T STARTED WITH FRED VINCY NOT FEELING WELL. Following a trip to the Houndsley horse fair, Fred had spent two days putting off his ailment as 'mere depression and headache'. When things took a turn for the worse on the third day, the Vincys sent for their old family doctor, who spoke of a 'slight derangement' before 'sending the usual white parcels' of medicine with 'black and drastic contents'. These did not help. At breakfast the next morning, Fred 'succeeded in nothing but in sitting and shivering by the fire'. Fortunately, it was at this moment that Fred's sister, Rosamond, happened to see the young Dr Lydgate pass through Lowick Gate. Ignoring the feverish protests of her son, Fred's mother sprang to the window and, 'thinking only of Fred and not of medical etiquette', asked Dr Lydgate to come in. Lydgate's diagnosis was as clear as it was terrifying: 'he was convinced that Fred was in the pink-skinned stage of typhoid fever, and that he had taken just the wrong medicines. He must go to bed immediately, must have a regular nurse, and various appliances and precautions must be used.'[1]

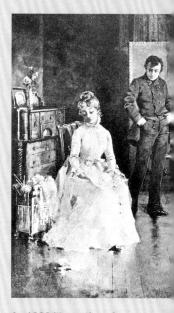

An 1888 illustration of *Middlemarch*, showing an encounter between Dr Lydgate and Rosamond Vincy – Fred's sister.

Of course, Lydgate had no way of being sure of his diagnosis. Having studied in Paris, he had only recently read the great French anatomist Pierre-Charles-Alexandre Louis's study of the subtle pathological differences between typhus and typhoidal (typhus-like) fevers. However, without conducting an autopsy on the still very much alive Fred Vincy, Lydgate only had a fever and a pink rash to go on, which were 'very equivocal in its beginnings'.[1] Neither could he be sure that his prescribed course of rest, diet and tonics would work.

In the absence of any specific treatment, all one could do was hope for the best and pray that the infection would not spread to others. When Fred's father came home, he was very angry: 'It was no joke to have fever in the house. Everybody must be sent to now, not to come to dinner on Thursday. And [the family servant] Pritchard needn't get up any wine: brandy was the best thing against infection.' The younger Vincy children were evacuated 'to a farmhouse the morning after Fred's illness had declared itself'. In the event, everything ended well. After spending several days in a delirium, Fred 'became simply feeble', and the neighbours no 'longer considered the house in quarantine'.[1] Meanwhile, the frequent encounters between Dr Lydgate and Rosamond at Fred's bedside gave rise first to feelings of respect, and soon much more than that ...

Published between 1871 and 1872, this fictional yet strikingly intimate account of typhoid fever in Mary Ann Evans's (pen name George Eliot) novel Middlemarch highlights the terrifying, mystifying and everyday nature of the disease in Victorian England. Typhoid fever is caused by the rod-shaped bacterium *Salmonella enterica* serovar Typhi (hereafter *S.* Typhi). *S.* Typhi passes invisibly from human to human in contaminated water and food. If untreated, it can kill up to one in five of those it infects. Survivors may still suffer from debilitating long-term damage to their intestine. By the time Middlemarch was published, typhoid was a familiar scourge. For centuries, typhoid and related enteric fevers had claimed a steady and grim toll on human lives and health across the world. The disease posed a particular threat to city dwellers, armies and survivors of major catastrophes, who often had no access to clean water. Although the poor were at greater risk of contracting it, typhoid's victims also included royalty, presidents and the rich and famous.[2] [3] [4]

Much of this was about to change. Unbeknownst to Mary Ann Evans and the fictional inhabitants of *Middlemarch*, the next 150 years would see humans develop an impressive arsenal of ways to prevent, diagnose and treat typhoid. Thanks to sophisticated sanitation systems, microbiological surveillance and hygiene protocols, along with vaccines and antibiotics, most people reading these pages will never encounter typhoid. Instead, they will read about it in Victorian novels as a vanquished threat from a bygone era, or perhaps briefly think of it when they receive their travel vaccinations ahead of a holiday. And yet typhoid is far from dead. According to current estimates, *S*. Typhi still sickens between 11 million and 20 million people, and kills between 120,000 and 161,000 people every year.[5] What is more, the bacterium is becoming resistant to the drugs we use to treat it. Over the past three decades, the international spread of a new genetic variant of *S*. Typhi has triggered a gathering storm of antibiotic-resistant typhoid outbreaks. Although there is hope in the form of next-generation typhoid conjugate vaccines, decades of efforts to control this ancient disease hang in the balance.[6]

How could it come to this situation, and how can analysing past control efforts make current interventions more effective? Building on the award-winning *Typhoidland* exhibitions,[6] this book engages with these questions by exploring two hundred years of typhoid control through the eyes of everyday people and the experts devising new interventions. Part One introduces readers to typhoid's biology and evolutionary history. Part Two shows how the nineteenth century saw key advances in our understanding of the ways bacterial pathogens spread. Part Three focuses on the well-known English university town of Oxford as a case study to reveal how Victorian engineers, epidemiologists and campaigners used fears of typhoid to push for investment in sanitation and water supply infrastructure. It also discusses how desperate doctors and patients looked for effective treatments and how scientists used new knowledge of typhoid's bacterial cause to develop vaccines and drugs – but also had to battle against vaccine opposition – occasionally resorting to dubious trial methods. Finally, Part Four highlights how poverty, neglect and false tropes of typhoid as a disease of the past have contributed to a dangerous loss of international control. While this is no academic monograph, what follows is based on rigorous research, with references pointing to further literature. Hopefully, readers will enjoy reading this book, come to appreciate our shared human history of typhoid and realise that – as with so many other infectious diseases – progress depends less on individual moments of genius than on sustained solidarity.

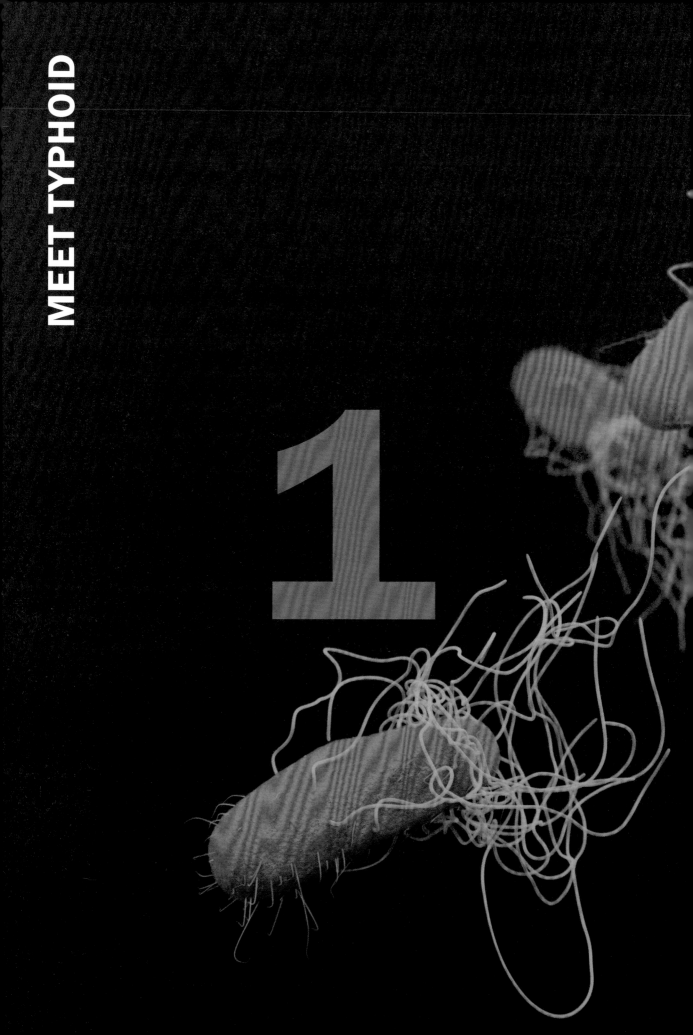

1

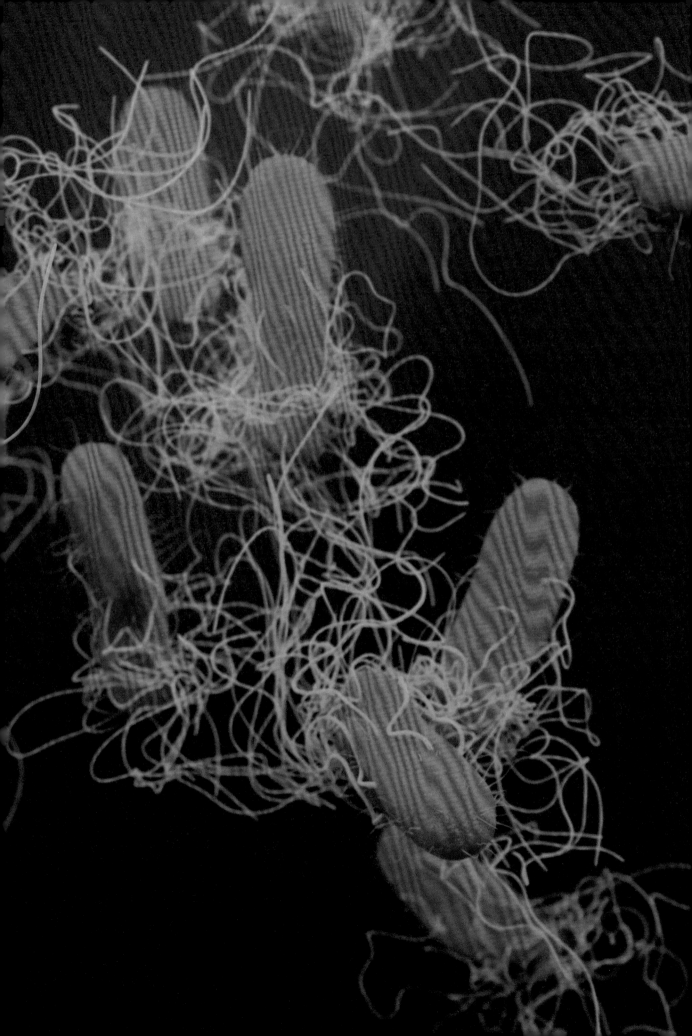

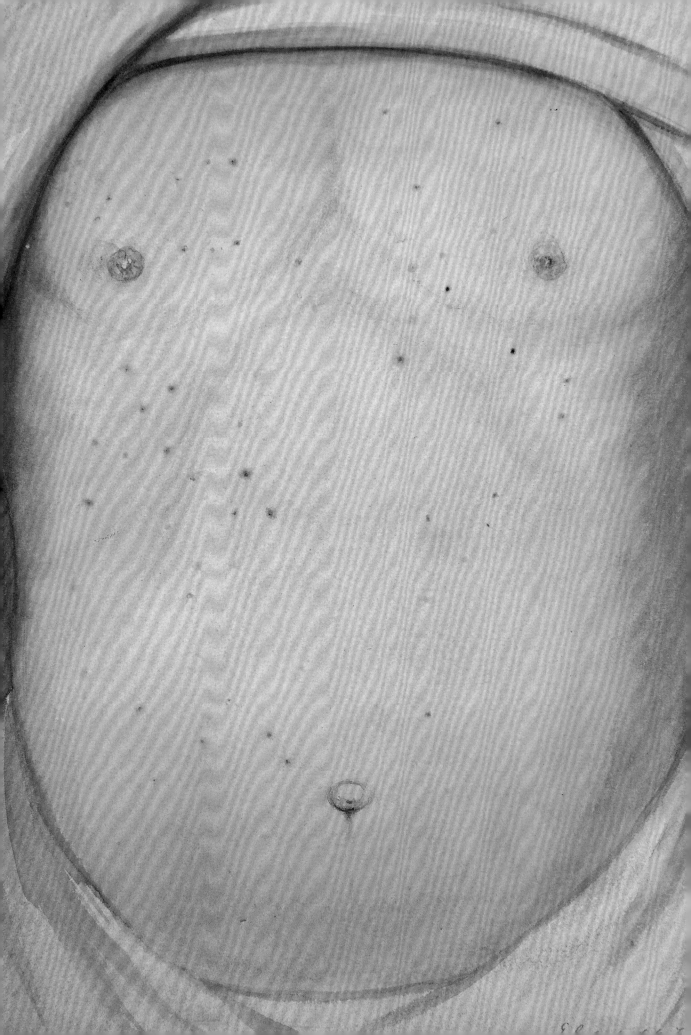

CHAPTER TWO

The biology and evolution of a major killer

Unseen by Alice and her friends, [the river] contained a germ.
It was small, rod-shaped and hairy.
Its name is typhoid and this is its story.

ALICE IN TYPHOIDLAND, 2020

S ALMONELLA ENTERICA serovar Typhi – or *S.* Typhi – the bacterial cause of typhoid, is a distinct species within the large group (genus) of *Salmonella* microbes. After departing from a common ancestor that they shared with *Escherichia coli* bacteria, *Salmonella* bacteria spent millions of years co-evolving with their animal hosts, which include birds, reptiles, amphibians and mammals. To survive, they had to develop an ever-expanding array of tools to overcome their hosts' immune defences and outcompete other organisms. Over time, evolution in the form of mutations and the 'horizontal' exchange of beneficial genes with other bacteria gave rise to distinct new *Salmonella* species and types. While most *Salmonella* continued to infect a large number of animal hosts, some carved out a niche by specialising in only one host species. In the case of *S.* Typhi, this host was the human species.[8]–[11]

When this so-called host restriction took place is unclear. Over the past three decades, researchers have developed sophisticated methods to reconstruct the genetic history of organisms by comparing the number of mutations in the form of single-nucleotide polymorphisms (SNPs) in different samples. Put simply, the more SNPs an organism has acquired relative to another, the more distant they are on the so-called phylogenetic tree of related organisms. While SNPs tell us about the relative position of an organism on a phylogenetic tree, it is not possible to say exactly when they occurred without further contextual archaeological or ancient DNA evidence. By assuming an approximately constant rate of molecular evolution, researchers believed that they might be able to use 'molecular clocks' to come to more precise temporal estimates of the emergence of *S.* Typhi, and dated it to roughly 10,000 to 43,000 years ago.[8] However, subsequent findings of rapid genetic evolution during outbreaks and external selection pressure has led to an abandonment of this molecular clock approach.[9] [12]

Regardless of when typhoid emerged, its highly specialised mode of spreading made it ideally suited

OPPOSITE
Thomas Godard, chest and abdomen of a patient with unusually copious typhoid eruptions, late nineteenth-century watercolour.

RIGHT
A photomicrograph of *Salmonella enterica* serovar Typhi – the bacterial cause of typhoid fever – using a Gram-stain technique, 1979.

to increasingly dense human settlement patterns. S. Typhi enters the body in contaminated water and food. Although the bacterium is capable of surviving the gastric acid in our stomachs, successful infection of a new host depends on exposure to relatively large numbers of bacteria.[13] Once S. Typhi bacteria have attached to the mucosal layer of the small intestine, they make their way to the inner submucosal region of the small bowel, either by tricking specialised local immune cells (lymphoid epithelial M-Cells) to carry them across, or by squeezing in-between the gut epithelial cells. Once through, bacteria begin to multiply in the inner submucosal region of the small bowel and can cause excessive tissue growth (hypertrophy) in a particular area of the small intestine called Peyer's patches – named after seventeenth-century Swiss anatomist Johann Conrad Peyer. These patches can die (necrose), which is believed to be a cause of ileal perforation, a potentially fatal complication of typhoid. From the hypertrophied Peyer's patches, S. Typhi make the jump into the human bloodstream and lymphatic system. They then begin to multiply within the reticuloendothelial system, which consists of cells (macrophages) involved with the body's immune response. Special proteins on S. Typhi's surface (antigens) allow the bacteria to reside in immune cells such as macrophages, and to survive in the liver, spleen and bone marrow.[14]

Initially, typhoid victims are not aware that they are carrying and excreting typhoid bacteria. It is only after an asymptomatic period of between seven to fourteen days that some – but not necessarily all – victims show distinct clinical

S. Typhi is part of the large group (genus) of *Salmonella* microbes. *Salmonella* bacteria spent millions of years co-evolving with their animal hosts, which include birds, reptiles, amphibians and mammals. S. Typhi is the result of a distinct evolutionary branch that produced a highly specialised obligate pathogen that only infects humans and cannot survive for long outside the human body.

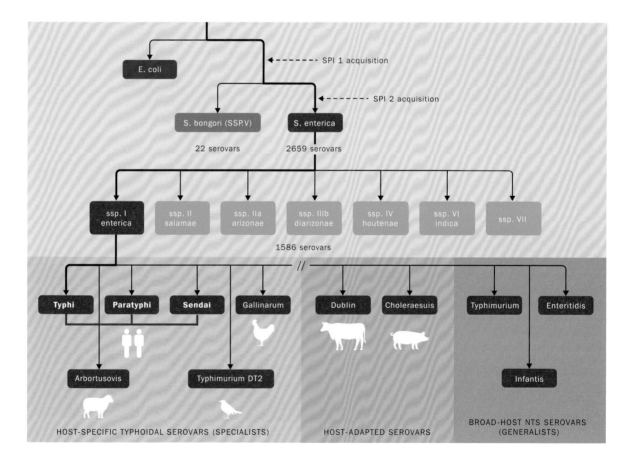

symptoms of a typhoid infection. Symptoms that occur can range from fever to abdominal symptoms, including pain, nausea, vomiting, constipation or diarrhoea. As the disease progresses, some patients go on to develop a characteristic rose-coloured rash, while others develop intermittent confusion and become apathetic.[15] In the worst cases, victims may die as a result of complications resulting from gastrointestinal haemorrhage, intestinal perforation and typhoid encephalopathy. Relapses can occur after the end of the first fever.[14]

While S. Typhi can kill up to one in five of its victims, its most successful evolutionary strategy rests in the ability to permanently establish itself in the gall bladders and – less often – urinary tracts of between one to five per cent of typhoid survivors.[11] So-called chronic carriers of typhoid, such as the (in)famous cook 'Typhoid Mary' Mallon (see Chapter 9), show no outward sign of infection, but intermittently excrete large numbers of S. Typhi in their stool or urine – from where they can go on to silently infect new hosts.

K.H. Baumgärtner, portrait of a patient with progressed typhoid fever, from *Kranken-Physiognomik*, 1929.

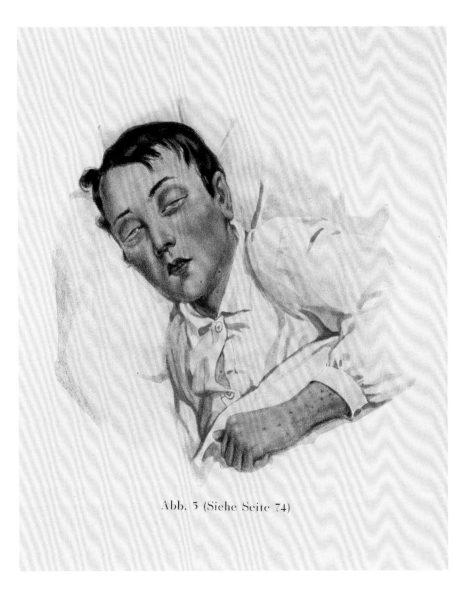

Abb. 3 (Siehe Seite 74)

FIND TYPHOID

from autopsy to bacteriology

2

Distinguishing typhoid fever from other diseases is difficult without access to modern diagnostics and laboratories. Some enteric diseases that affect the intestine, such as cholera, frequently occur in explosive waves, with victims suffering from easily recognisable symptoms like 'rice water' diarrhoea, and a distinctive purple-bluish hue resulting from acute dehydration.[16] By contrast, the symptoms of typhoid fever are more varied, and are easy to confuse with other diseases, such as malaria or typhus, which also cause fever, rashes, diarrhoea and dehydration. It is therefore no surprise that typhoid outbreaks were historically often described using the generic term 'fever', and lumped together with other diseases. Although older sources speak of a variety of typhus-like (or typhoidal) fevers,[17] it was only in the nineteenth century that researchers began to isolate and create the modern disease category of typhoid from the wider background noise of infectious fevers. This was not a straightforward process. Instead, it involved different ways of finding typhoid: first in the body, then in the environment and finally under the microscope and in the blood.

OPPOSITE
An early visualisation of the innate immune response. 'The battle in a drop of blood – white cells breaking up the typhoid fever parasite: Health & Disease in Deadly Combat', c.1900.

TYPHUS ABDOMINALIS. NECROSIS SUPERFICIAL

Gezeichnet von W. GUMMELT.

VERLAG UND CHROMOGRAPHIE DER KUNSTANSTALT (vorm. GUSTAV W. SEITZ) A.-G. WANDSBEK

CHAPTER THREE

Typhoid inside the body

'Of all these lesions only one was constantly found, namely an alteration of the elliptical patches of the small intestine, to which may be added a morbid change in the mesenteric glands. I have considered it as inseparable from the disease we are now studying, and as absolutely forming its anatomical characteristic.'

PIERRE-CHARLES-ALEXANDRE LOUIS, 1829
[1835 TRANSLATION] VOL. I, 381–384[22]

OUR MODERN concept of typhoid fever as a distinct clinical disease emerged in fits and starts between the 1820s and 1850s. Key to this development was a twin revolution. Across Europe and North America, a young generation of medical researchers was becoming dissatisfied with existing disease theories' lack of specificity. Radicalised by an age of revolution, they strove to develop a new 'rational' approach to studying fevers and other maladies by linking symptoms to pathological changes in the body and using statistics to show that these links were due to more than coincidence.

Born in Ay, Champagne, two years ahead of the French Revolution in 1787, the French physician Pierre-Charles-Alexandre Louis – whom we first encountered being referred to in *Middlemarch* – was a typical example of this new generation. After initially training in law, Louis studied medicine in Reims and Paris. During his training, Louis would have been exposed to the groundbreaking works on probability by English statistician Thomas Bayes and on statistical correlation by French mathematician Pierre-Simon Laplace. In Paris, he would also have encountered a new form of systematised pathological investigation, which saw anatomists and physiologists at the famous Hôtel Dieu hospital study diseases as distinct and localised conditions that began in specific tissues. Both concepts would have a profound influence on Louis.

Previous generations had conceived of disease as resulting from hydrological imbalances of the four Galenic humours (blood, yellow and black bile, and phlegm) or from nervous overstimulation or understimulation. These imbalances could be caused by a variety of factors including patients' lifestyles or external factors like bad weather or putrid air. Practitioners tried to rectify these imbalances with tailored diets, bloodletting, purging, by removing patients from 'unhealthy' climates, or by using stimulants and depressants.[18] [19]

Louis graduated in 1813, and his experience of practising medicine in Odessa, in modern-day Ukraine, made him sceptical of these generalised disease theories and resulting treatments. Around 1820, he returned to Paris and began to work at the city's large Hôpital de la Charité, where he embarked on a research programme to

OPPOSITE
An illustration of *Typhus Abdominalis* (typhoid fever) showing necrosis of intestine by Alfred Kast, 1892–95.

distinguish between fevers and to uncover potential causes and effective treatments. Key to Louis's endeavour was studying fevers in a large number of patients and using statistical methods to analyse his results. Over the next six years, he recorded over 2,000 case histories and autopsy results. Using his case notes, Louis began to differentiate between fevers by statistically linking the occurrence of specific organ damages to a set of defined symptoms. He also 'averaged out' groups of patients suffering from the same disease to determine whether treatments worked, while also taking into account factors such as age, severity of disease and diet.[19] [20]

Use of what later became known as the *méthode numerique* allowed Louis to promote a shift in medical thinking about fevers. Published in 1825, his *Recherches anatomo-patholgiques et thérapeutiques sur la phthisie* not only challenged concepts of fever resulting from a generalised inflammation of the organs, but also confirmed the specificity of tuberculosis as a distinct disease.[20] [21] Louis next applied the same method to continued fevers in other parts of the body. He soon found that one common type of fever was characterised in life by diarrhoea and rose-coloured spots on the abdomen and after death by lesions on the Peyer's patches in the small intestine.* In 1829, Louis published his results in two volumes with the lengthy title *Recherches anatomiques, pathologiques et thérapeutiques sur la maladie connue sous les noms de gastroentérite, fièvre putride, adynamique, ataxique, typhoïde, etc.* [19]–[22]

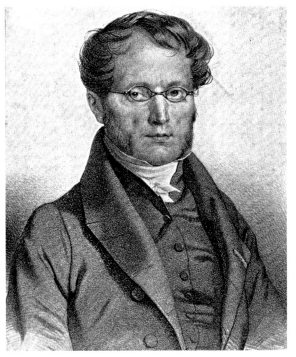

Pierre-Charles-Alexandre Louis coined the term typhoid fever in 1829.

Reactions to Louis's work were varied. Many physicians remained convinced that fevers resulted from general inflammation or humoural imbalances. Others distrusted the novel statistical reasoning Louis was employing. In Britain, physicians noted that they had been unable to find the Peyer's patch lesions Louis had described in victims of 'true' or 'British typhus',** which was common in the country's industrialising towns, and whose fever curve closely matched that of typhoid. In the newly independent United States, most physicians were interested less in continuous fevers like typhoid and more in the periodic malarial fevers that were common along the east coast. Some, however, noted that the 'continued fever' of New England, which often was given the adjective 'typhous' to signify similarity to typhus, nonetheless seemed to be distinct from British descriptions of 'true' typhus fever.[21]

---

* Louis was not the only person to report that a certain kind of fever led to lesions on the Peyer's patches. In the French city of Tours, medical officer Pierre Bretonneau coined the condition dothienenenteritis (boil of the intestine) after conducting autopsies on victims of regional fever outbreaks around 1820.[17]

** During the early 19th century, large fever outbreaks (variously described as Irish Fever or True British Typhus) occurred among Irish emigrants and poorer population segments on both sides of the Atlantic. Although it is impossible to be certain, is likely that these outbreaks were due to louse-borne epidemic typhus (*Rickettsia prowazekii*) and not to typhoid fever (*S. Typhi*).[23]

Three American researchers who were interested in finding ways of differentiating between these fevers were Enoch Hale and James Jackson at Boston's Massachusetts General Hospital and William Wood Gerhard at the Pennsylvania Hospital in Philadelphia. Mirroring a wider shift of US training towards French methods, both Jackson and Gerhard had studied under Louis in Paris. Investigations in Boston soon ground to a halt: Hale only published a brief observation on differences between 'typhus' and 'typhous' fevers in 1833, and Jackson died before completing a French-style anatomical-statistical investigation in 1834. Encouraged by Gerhard in Philadelphia, Jackson's father nonetheless published his son's preliminary investigations in 1835. Gerhard published his own observations in the same year. Between 1833 and 1835, he had applied Louis's methodology and systematically looked for Peyer's patches lesions during post-mortem examinations of fever cases at the Pennsylvania Hospital. Both Jackson and Gerhard's findings indicated that the continued fever of New England was the same as Louis's typhoid fever, and that the disease was distinct from periodic malarial fevers. One year later, a severe winter outbreak of typhus in Philadelphia, with over 2,000 cases in poorer neighbourhoods, allowed Gerhard and another Louis pupil, Caspar Pennock, to establish that typhoid fever was also non-identical with typhus fever.[21]

Although Gerhard and Pennock's observations were disputed by others, the following decades saw a growing number of influential physicians begin to distinguish between typhoid and other fevers. Perhaps most importantly, the new clinical-anatomical definition of typhoid was adopted by University College London pathologist and future royal physician William Jenner (1815–1898). Between 1847 and 1849, Jenner conducted a mammoth symptomatic and pathological study of continued fever at London's Fever Hospital. Using Louis's *méthode numérique*, Jenner not only re-confirmed the pathological distinction between typhus and typhoid, but also claimed to be able to distinguish between both diseases in life due to the characteristic rose spots caused by typhoid and the different rash caused by typhus. Moving from the clinic to the field, Jenner also traced fever cases back to the houses in which they originated. His research showed that typhus and typhoid patients came from different households, and that an increase or decrease in the number of cases caused by one fever did not affect the prevalence of the other.[3] [21] [24]

Jenner's mix of anatomical, statistical and field study approaches not only made him Britain's leading typhoid expert, but also brought him into contact with royalty.[3] As a freshly appointed Physician Extraordinary to Queen Victoria, the fourth son of a Kent innkeeper was hastily summoned to Windsor Castle in late November 1861 to attend to the 42-year-old Prince Consort. Albert had a long history of gastrointestinal issues, which had been exacerbated by taking on additional government duties. Things had taken a turn for the worse in summer 1861, following the scandalous affair of Albert's son, the Prince of Wales, with Irish actress Nellie Clifden. When rumours surfaced that the prince was still involved with Clifden, Albert travelled to Cambridge on 25 November to resolve the situation. On his return, Albert was fatigued and suffering from back and leg pains. Jenner and fellow Royal Physician Sir James Clark soon suspected typhoid fever, but waited for the characteristic rose spots to reveal themselves between the eighth and twelfth day of

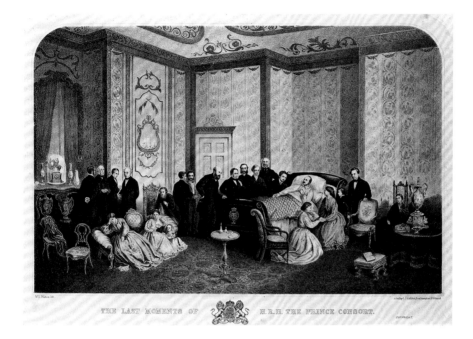

THE LAST MOMENTS OF H.R.H. THE PRINCE CONSORT.

the acute disease. When a pink rash appeared on Saturday 7 December, Jenner made the diagnosis of typhoid fever. Although all four attending physicians maintained a determinedly optimistic outlook, Albert's health deteriorated rapidly. On 14 December, the Prince Consort died.[25] According to his wife, Queen Victoria, his departure was peaceful:

> '...the breathing was the alarming thing – so rapid, I think 60 respirations in a minute... He seemed half dozing, quite quiet... I left the room for a moment and sat down on the floor in utter despair. Attempts at consolation from others only made me worse...Alice told me to come in...and I took his dear left hand which was already cold, though the breathing was quite gentle and I knelt down by him...Two or three long but perfectly gentle breaths were drawn, the hand clasping mine and... all, all was over.' [26]

Although Albert's official cause of death was given as typhoid fever, some modern writers speculate that his long-standing health issues indicate an alternative, underlying cause of death.[27] [28] This goes against the clinical judgement of William Jenner, who was one of the leading typhoid experts of his time, and also against the views of the three other senior physicians attending the Prince Consort. Ultimately, the fact that no diagnostic tests existed and that no autopsy was conducted makes it impossible to know which mix of underlying and immediate causes killed Albert, and if Jenner might have confused the symptoms he had studied so intensively.

Rather than indulging in retrospective diagnosis, what is far more revealing about the death of one of the most powerful and wealthy men of his time is how little was still known about typhoid fever in 1861. Thirty-two years after Louis's description of necrosed Peyer's patches, the cause and spread of typhoid fever remained mysterious. Developing effective preventive measures would depend on translating anatomical observations of typhoid lesions in one body into ways of tracing the disease's spread from body to body.

Death of the Prince Consort, c. 1865. The Prince Consort lies in bed, and Queen Victoria sits on his left. In a group on the far left stand the prince's physicians: Sir William Jenner, Sir James Clark, Sir Henry Holland and Sir Thomas Watson.

CHAPTER FOUR

Typhoid
outside the body

The sewer may be looked upon, in fact, as a direct
continuation of the diseased intestine.
WILLIAM BUDD, 1856[29]

THE FOUNDATIONS for a new mode of tracing the spread of infectious
disease had already been laid by the time Albert died. Although attempts
to map disease date back hundreds of years,[30] the mid-nineteenth
century saw a growing number of countries and enterprising research-
ers start to gather data on disease – not just at the local level, but also nationally and
in colonial territories. Underlying this surge of data collection was the spread of
statistical literacy, growing state interest in surveying the health and efficiency of
domestic and colonial populations, and the multiple collective panics caused by
cholera pandemics, which swept the globe from the 1820s onwards.[31]

Administrators and budding public health experts used the new data sets, door-
to-door investigations and epidemiological research on institutionalised, enslaved
and non-European colonial populations to study outbreak dynamics. They also
looked for correlations between disease incidence and conducive environmental,
climatic, 'constitutional' and socioeconomic factors. Resulting statistical analyses,
maps and field investigations revealed previously unknown links. They also
connected provincial and colonial medical practitioners with metropolitan public
health workers, and were wielded to argue for competing interpretations of how a
disease occurred as well as investment in preventive measures.[3]

European nation states were at the forefront of this new age of disease
conceptualisation. During an era of rapid industrialisation, imperial expansion and
urbanisation, concerns about social unrest and revolutionary upheaval saw ruling
elites agree to major reforms of existing welfare and administrative systems. The
wider context of reform created opportunities for a new generation of medically
trained and numerically capable experts to press for a mix of social and public
health-oriented interventions.[23] [32]–[34]

In Britain, sanitary reformers such as Thomas Southwood Smith and Edwin
Chadwick, who were strongly influenced by the utilitarian philosophy of Jeremy
Bentham, published studies linking disease incidence to poverty and inadequate
sanitation. Chadwick, in particular, played a key role in focusing domestic British
politics on questions of sanitation. His famous 1842 *Report on the Sanitary Condition
of the Labouring Population of Great Britain* prompted upgrades of London's sewage
and water supply infrastructure, and encouraged the British government to pass its
first Public Health Act, in 1848. Chadwick's efforts were complemented by those of
the statistician William Farr. Born in 1807, Farr had studied medicine in Paris,
attended lectures by Louis (Chapter 3), and subsequently worked as compiler of
abstracts within the newly founded General Register Office (GRO). As part of this

CHOLERA MORBUS.

The best means of avoiding this dreadful disease are,

1. Fresh Air, as much as possible ; only taking care not to catch cold.
2. To be cleanly in the Skin, in the Clothes, in the House and round about it.
3. To lead a regular and sober life.—*Drunkards are among the first attacked, and likeliest to die.* Take plenty of exercise.
4. To keep a cheerful mind, never giving way to a dread of the disease.
5. Take no sour Food or Drink : use sparingly green Vegetables.

The First Signs of the Complaint are,

Giddiness in the Head. Sick Stomach. Shivering or Trembling all over. Great Coldness of the Skin. Low Pulse. General Weaknes. A Face as of one Dying. Cramp, beginning in the Toes and Fingers, and so spreading all over the Body.

The First Things to be done for those who are taken ill.

1. Put into a warm Bed, and put several hot dry Blankets over.
2. Send directly for the Doctor ;—much depends on his speedy help.
3. Give to drink, once every hour, a quarter of a pint of hot Water, with a table-spoonful of Kitchen Salt in it, until a quantity of dark stuff is brought up from the Stomach—then
4. Give to drink, weak hot Brandy and Water, with Ginger or Peppermint.
5. Rub the Body with hot Flannel.
6. Poultice the Feet, Legs, and Stomach, with equal parts of Mustard and Oatmeal.
7. Keep the Body warm all over with hot bags of Bran or Sand.—Worsted Stockings would do for Bags.
8. In very bad cases, or if the Doctor should be long in coming, give from 20 to 40 drops of Laudanum in the hot Brandy and Water ; but be sure to count the Drops.

KEEP THIS PAPER,

For your Direction, in case the Cholera should break out in the Parish; and in the mean time, WITHOUT DELAY, take the following Precautions :—

1. Keep your House clean and well aired. Open the Windows daily.
2. Clear out all Drains and Ditches near you, and take away all heaps of Filth from near your Houses.
3. Keep your Families as clean, and feed them as well as you possibly can ; and clothe them comfortably warm.
4. Be sure to lead a regular & sober Life.
5. Get your House white-washed with hot Lime, without Delay.

THE CHOLERA MORBUS is a deadly plague, by means of which Almighty God has cut off *Hundreds of Thousands* of mankind in foreign parts. It has now reached this country, and has killed upwards of *Fifteen Thousand* people after a few hours' illness. It is our duty to prevent, by all means in our power, its increase among ourselves, to preserve our own lives and those of our neighbours. For this end, it is very needful to keep the mind free from alarm. Now there is no way so sure of warding off the fear of death, as the answer of a good conscience towards God, and the hope of forgiveness and life eternal, through Jesus Christ our Lord. I entreat, therefore, your earnest attention to the few plain Rules which follow. Examine yourself thus :—

1. Am I now fit to die? Have I a good ground of hope to be saved through Jesus Christ. 2. Cor. xiii 5.
2. Do I hate all sin because it is hateful to God, and brought my Saviour to the Cross?
3. Have I a lively faith in God's mercy through Christ, with a thankful remembrance of His most precious death, and a lively hope of His eternal joy? Mark xi. 22. Heb. xi. 6.
4. Repent heartily of whatever you know you have done wrong ; repent heartily before God. Mark i. 15.
5. Amend your life, without delay, striving steadfastly to be more pure, sober, contented, humble, kind-hearted to your fellow creatures, holy, heavenly-minded. James iv. 8, Romans xiii. 11. 12.
6. Read daily in God's Holy Word, which alone, through the teaching of his Holy Spirit, can instruct you in His will, and make you wise unto salvation. John v. 39. Psalm xci.
7. Pray, therefore, daily, for God's Holy Spirit ; more especially on the Lord's Day, and in His House. Pray from the heart. And for your help herein, I entreat you to use, in private and in your family, the prayer which follows.

THE PRAYER.

O, ALMIGHTY GOD, who hast visited the Nations near us with the sudden death of thousands, turn away, we beseech Thee, from this thy favoured land, the wrath, which to our sins is justly due. Awaken us to repentance, whilst we have yet time. Make us to remember, that in the midst of life we are in death; and so teach us to number our days, that we may apply our hearts unto wisdom.

Humbly *I* confess, that in the pride and hardness of *my* heart, *I* have shewn *myself* unmindful of thy past mercies, and have followed unthankfully *my* own evil will, instead of thy most righteous laws. Give *me*, by thy Holy Spirit, true repentance. Make *me* to feel that *I* have destroyed myself by *my* sins, and that in Christ is *my* only help and hope. Thus may *I* obtain to-day, through his merits and sufferings, that forgiveness which to-morrow it may be too late to ask.

Strengthen *me* with might by thy Spirit in the inner man against the power of sin, and the dread of death. Give *me* a new and clean heart, that *I* may love, and fear, and obey thee in all *my* thoughts, words, and actions. Grant that in reading thy word *I* may grow daily in faith and holiness; that so, however soon *my* time may come, *I* may give up *my* soul into thy hands, O gracious Father, in the hope of life eternal, through our only Mediator, Jesus Christ the Lord.

work, Farr not only implemented an ambitious programme of data collection that linked demography and public health, but also published on the bell-curved regularity of expanding and contracting epidemics.[23] [33] [35]

Although data collection remained hampered by incomplete and inconsistent reporting, emerging mortality statistics and epidemiological investigations lent weight to long-standing concerns about water as an important element in the spread of infectious disease. When the third cholera pandemic hit the British Isles between 1848 and the 1850s, water-related concerns reached an early crescendo. Although practitioners engaged in vehement disagreements over whether cholera was caused by filth, poisons, noxious miasmatic air or a combination of such factors, many agreed that contaminated and stagnant water played a role in facilitating the spread of the much-feared disease.[3] [30]

Depending on their favoured transmission model, public health advocates employed different methods to highlight various water-related risk factors and argue for corresponding preventive interventions. Following the death of around 7,500 Londoners from cholera between September 1848 and August 1849, William Farr used mortality statistics to argue that elevation and citizens' relative distance from air-polluting filth and stagnant water was the primary determinant of health. It followed that improving water flows and reducing exposure to noxious gases would help prevent cholera. Fellow London physician John Snow came to different conclusions. In 1849, Snow had already suspected that cholera was spread not by inhaling tainted air, but by swallowing water contaminated with some kind of particulate matter or possibly living organism. Combining a painstaking house-to-house enquiry, a statistical analysis of case incidence data and skilful epidemiological mapping, Snow argued that an 1854 cholera outbreak in the environment of London's Broad Street was caused by something in the water that was acting on the alimentary tract. People who had consumed water supplied by the Southwark & Vauxhall and the Lambeth water companies, which drew their water directly from the Thames, had been particularly likely to contract cholera.[3] [23] [30] [33]

Now the stuff of many myths, Snow's monocausal water-focused theory of disease transmission was radical, and only gradually came to be accepted by the public health establishment – including Farr.* His efforts also did little to curb an already declining outbreak – and he never claimed to have removed the Broad Street pump handle.[37] Nonetheless, his combination of shoe-leather epidemiology, which involved door-to-door case tracking, quantitative methods and skilful use of maps to argue his case, was indicative of a new style of public health investigation that attempted to link pathologies in individual bodies to different environmental factors.[3] [23] [30] [33]

OPPOSITE
Starting around 1820, the terror caused by the cholera pandemics provided important momentum for a new mode of public health politics. This pamphlet combines a call for prayer with health advice designed to prevent 'Cholera Morbus' (London, c.1830s–40s).

* One of Snow's first converts was the assistant curate Henry Whitehead, who had conducted a detailed parallel door-to-door investigation of the Broad Street outbreak.[36]

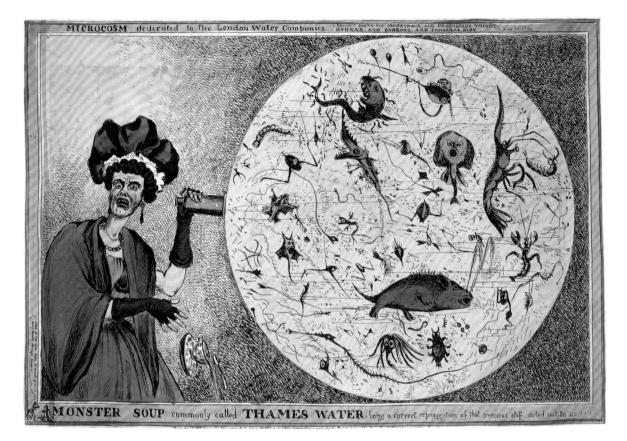

MICROCOSM dedicated to the London Water Companies. BROUGHT FORTH ALL MONSTROUS, ALL PRODIGIOUS THINGS, HYDRAS AND GORGONS, AND CHIMERAS DIRE. Vide Milton.

MONSTER SOUP commonly called THAMES WATER. being a correct representation of that precious stuff doled out to us !!!

Crucially, cholera was not the only disease to which this mix of methods was being applied. In the shadow of the pandemic, other investigators were beginning to draw similar conclusions regarding typhoid. In Bristol, physician William Budd had long suspected a link between typhoid and contaminated water. Having also studied under Louis in Paris, Budd had suffered a near fatal attack of typhoid fever while serving on the naval hospital ship HMS *Dreadnought* in 1838. His experience as a physician had long convinced him that typhoid was contagious when he had the opportunity to conduct a detailed study of typhoid transmission during an 1847 outbreak in Bristol's Clifton neighbourhood. Of the 34 households on Richmond Terrace, 13 had reported at least one case of typhoid. The one thing that separated these households from the 21 unaffected households was that they all drew water from the same well.[38] Seven years later, Budd made similar observations about the spread of cholera while overseeing Bristol's water supplies. Employing the now familiar mix of epidemiological and statistical reasoning, he began to describe sewage systems as an 'extension of the diseased intestine', and advocated 'using chemical agents [such as chloride of lime] to destroy the infectious properties of contagious poisons' like typhoid and cholera.[29] [39]

It took Budd a long time to publish his observations. Although he taught his theory of waterborne typhoid and cholera transmission at Bristol University, it was only between 1856 and 1860 that he wrote it up for publication in *The Lancet*. Once they appeared in print, Budd's articles generated similar controversy to the earlier reports published by Snow.[3] [38] Interestingly, country practitioners were among

William Heath (under the pseudonym 'Paul Pry'), *Monster Soup in the Thames*, 1828 – a satirical engraving depicting early concepts of micro-organisms, featuring a disgusted woman using a microscope to gauge the quality of Thames water supplied by London water companies.

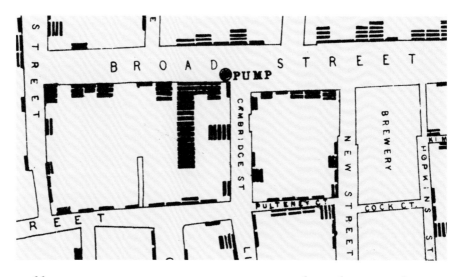

Detail of John Snow's 1854 visualisation of cholera incidence (each black line denotes an individual case) on Broad Street, with a depiction of the infamous pump.

Budd's strongest supporters. In contrast to metropolitan physicians, who were confronted with a host of interconnected disease environments, practitioners in regional cities or rural areas worked in less densely settled environments. This meant that they had greater opportunity to untangle how a disease might spread in a contagious manner between different households. Budd himself highlighted this 'better point of view'.[38] **

Another important source of support for Budd came from John Simon, who had started his public health career in London in 1848 and became Britain's longest-serving chief medical officer. From the 1860s onwards, Simon and his team of Medical Board investigators adopted Budd's waterborne theory of typhoid transmission and used a mix of disease statistics and epidemiological field investigations to press for sanitary reform throughout Britain. Moral argumentation was equally important. By presenting typhoid as a preventable 'filth disease', Simon turned typhoid incidence into a measure of civic virtue or shame.[3]

By the time Prince Albert died in December 1861, a growing number of – but by no means all – public health workers were thus arguing that typhoid spread in a contagionist manner in water and, as later investigations would show, also in contaminated food and milk. But even so-called contagionists still struggled to agree on what exactly caused typhoid. While some, like Budd, continued to talk of poisons that could spread by water and by air in confined spaces, others followed Snow in describing the causes of typhoid and cholera as particulate and possibly living matter. After finding evidence of typhoid during autopsies – and tracing its spread from human to human with statistics, maps and door-to-door epidemiology – uncovering and isolating the actual cause of typhoid was the next challenge. It was also a challenge that would slowly move typhoid research from the morgue, physician's practice and epidemiologist's office, to the bacteriologist's laboratory.

** Pierre Bretonneau (see p.16) [23] Henry Acland (see p.37) and Robert Koch (see p.52) also highlighted the value of less-populated rural areas for untangling typhoid epidemiology.

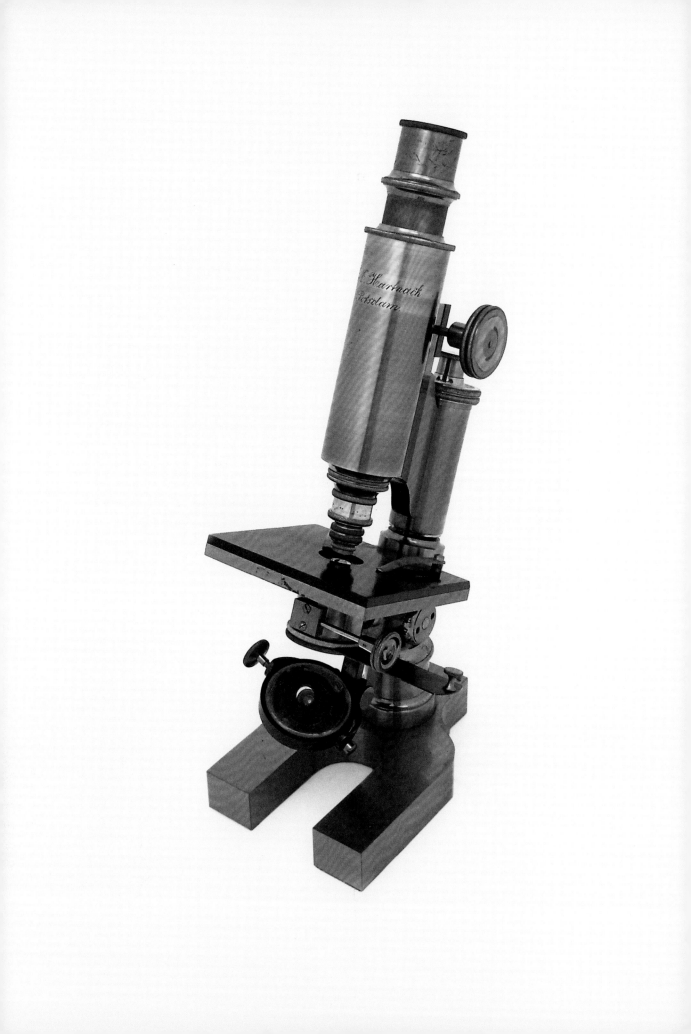

CHAPTER FIVE

Typhoid
under the microscope

In 23 cases, I encountered organisms 12 times ...
Where ... the heaps are less dense, which is the case in the
ray-like offshoots of the colonies, one can see at slightly
stronger magnification in the edges almost nothing
but rod-like entities ... The ends of them are rounded ...
Common to all is the soft contour ...

CARL JOSEPH EBERTH (AUTHOR TRANSLATION), 1880 [40]

THE FIRST CONFIRMED REPORT we have of a human coming face to face with typhoid's bacterial cause dates from late 1879, when, during the cold winter months, the Swiss city of Zurich experienced a major typhoid outbreak. In hospitals and homes across the city, patients suffered from fever and a range of abdominal symptoms, including pain, nausea, vomiting, constipation and diarrhoea. Of those who died, some were transported to the laboratory of German-born pathologist Carl Joseph Eberth. Sporting the giant bushy beard characteristic of many scholars of his generation, Eberth systematically analysed the corpses. He looked for the distinctive swelling and lesions within the Peyer's patch area, and took samples of the lower larynx, lymph nodes and spleen, which he prepared for bacteriological analysis on slides with acetic acid. Peering down his Parisian Hartnack microscope, he saw the rod-shaped bacterial cause of typhoid – *Salmonella enterica* serovar Typhi.[40]

Published in 1880, Eberth's drawing of typhoid's bacterial cause marked a personal triumph. It simultaneously formed part of a wider whirlwind of scientific reports on the isolation of the microbial causes of disease. Starting in the late 1850s and gathering steam during the 1860s and 1870s, a new school of microbiology had begun to systematically study how microorganisms impacted fermentation, agricultural production and human and animal health. With strong centres in Paris and Berlin, self-styled bacteriologists had employed a mix of microscopy, selective culturing and staining to identify, isolate and taxonomise different microorganisms. In addition to typhoid, the years around 1880 saw microbiologists identify further pathogens, such as *Bacillus anthracis* (anthrax) (1876), *Staphylococcus* (c.1878), *Neisseria gonorrhoeae* (gonorrhoea) and *Pasteurella multocida* (chicken cholera) (1879), *Streptococcus pneumoniae* (pneumonia and meningitis) (1881), *Mycobacterium tuberculosis*

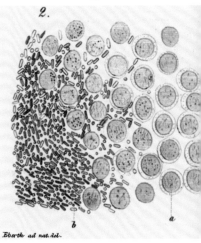

Eberth ad nat. del.

OPPOSITE
A Hartnack horseshoe-foot microscope (c.1886), similar to the type that was used by Carl Eberth to observe S. Typhi.

RIGHT
Carl Eberth's drawing of S. Typhi.[40]

(tuberculosis) (1882), *Corynebacterium diphtheriae* (diphtheria) and *Vibrio cholerae* (cholera) (1883), *Clostridium tetani* (tetanus) (1884) and *Meningococcus* (meningitis) (1887).[2] [4] [31] [41]

Reconciling different investigators' written descriptions and drawings of microbial organisms often proved challenging. To maintain the credibility of their discipline, and to resolve questions of priority during an age of intense nationalist scientific rivalry, microbiologists tried to supplement traditional reports with new modes of presenting evidence. In 1880, the school of German bacteriologists surrounding Robert Koch were already using photography to capture images of microscopic organisms. They were also developing what would become a four-step gold standard for the identification of a new pathogen ('Koch's Postulates'): finding an abundance of one microbe in an organism suffering from disease, isolating and growing this microbe on pure culture, successfully infecting an experimental organism with the suspected microbial pathogen and re-isolating this pathogen from the infected organism.[42]

Because Eberth had only completed the first step of this process, the small Berlin team surrounding Koch began work on isolating the suspected typhoid microbe. In 1881, Koch confirmed Eberth's observations and took the first photograph of what was then variously described as *Eberthella Typhi*, Eberth's bacillus or bacillus typhosus.[43]

The laborious work of isolating and growing (culturing) the microbe was left to Koch's pupil, the military physician and bacteriologist Georg Gaffky. To differentiate them from other bacteria, Gaffky first streaked human tissue containing the suspected typhoid bacteria onto nutrient gelatine plates and incubated the plates for 48 hours at room temperature. He then tried to select the bacteria he was interested in, replated and incubated this selection, and repeated this process until he had obtained a culture of *S.* Typhi that could be considered pure. Gaffky next developed additional culturing methods, including inoculating *S.* Typhi onto the surface of boiled potatoes to study colony formation, and experimented with solidified sheep blood serum, fluid serum and bouillon. However, he failed to isolate *S.* Typhi from victims' blood or faeces. He also failed to produce an experimental infection and reisolate *S.* Typhi from a whole menagerie of animals – the ultimate bacteriological proof, according to the famous Kochian postulates. Nonetheless, Gaffky was able to report that he had isolated and grown pure *S.* Typhi cultures from 26 of 28 confirmed typhoid fever cases in 1884.[44]

Gaffky's laboratory success capped a remarkable process of transformation for an initially very vaguely defined fever category. Just over half a century after Louis's description of Peyer's patch lesions, typhoid fever was now associated with a causative micro-organism, which could be observed, cultured and manipulated.

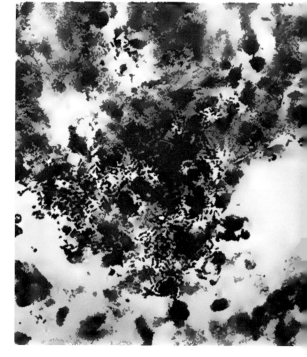

Robert Koch's photograph of *S.* Typhi, 1881.[43]

CHAPTER SIX

Typhoid
in the blood

Here is a simple and rapid process which can be employed by everyone, necessitating no laboratory material. All that is necessary is to have at one's disposal pure cultures of Eberth's bacillus, a microscope, and a few drops of serum or even only one drop of the blood of a patient.

FERNAND WIDAL, 1896[45]

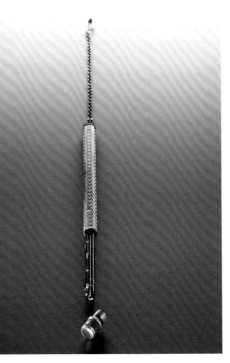

**Clinical thermometer,
c.1885–1900.**

INITIALLY, Eberth and Gaffky's laboratory breakthroughs changed little for day-to-day medical or public health practice (see Chapter 11). The new tenets of bacteriology were far from universally accepted.[46] Meanwhile, early difficulties in culturing S. Typhi from blood, water, food and faeces meant that the laboratory continued to play a subordinate role during outbreak investigations.[3] However, in the medium term, being able to culture S. Typhi opened the door for targeted biomedical interventions such as vaccines and diagnostics.

The need for improved typhoid diagnostics was particularly acute. Since the 1860s, advances in medical thermometry had aided the symptom-based diagnosis of typhoid fever. Armed with increasingly precise clinical thermometers, physicians such as Carl Wunderlich in Germany and Johns Hopkins University co-founder William Osler plotted the temperature curves of hundreds of patients and highlighted differences between fevers caused by malaria and those caused by typhoid. The curves aided bedside diagnosis and contemporary attempts to treat typhoid by lowering patients' temperature (Part Three). However, basing diagnosis on fever curves and rose spots alone remained imprecise, and required prolonged clinical observation, which was not possible in many settings.[47] [48]

In view of the limitations of clinical and culture-based diagnosis, a test was needed that could rapidly indicate whether or not a patient was infected with S. Typhi. Developing such a test became possible thanks to the twin emergence of the scientific disciplines of immunology (the study of the immune system) and serology (the study of serum – the fluid component of blood after blood cells and clotting factors have been removed).

By the 1880s, an increasing number of researchers were shifting from merely trying to identify pathogens to understanding what happened in a host after an initial infection. Key questions centred on understanding how pathogens spread and multiplied in the host's

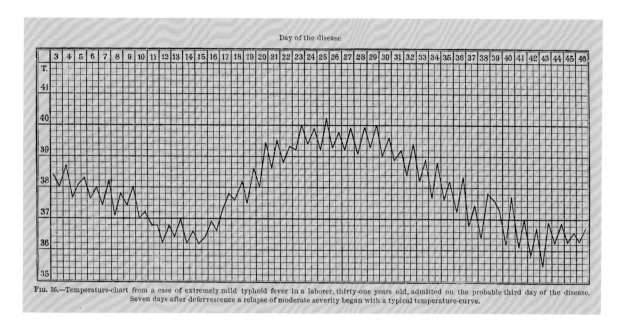

Day of the disease.

FIG. 36.—Temperature-chart from a case of extremely mild typhoid fever in a laborer, thirty-one years old, admitted on the probable third day of the disease. Seven days after defervescence a relapse of moderate severity began with a typical temperature-curve.

body, why some hosts seemed to be immune to infection, and how the growing number of new vaccines (Chapter 10) worked. Findings highlighted the complexity of the body's immune system.[49]

A c.1901 temperature chart depicting a mild case of typhoid in a 31-year-old labourer.

In 1882, Russian-born researcher Ilya – Élie – Metchnikoff observed that specialised cells – phagocytes – in the larvae of starfish could identify and attack foreign objects such as the thorns of a rose or tangerine tree. He soon observed similar cells in the blood of other animals and found that they could identify, engulf and eliminate invading fungal spores and bacteria. Phagocytes form part of the body's innate immune system, which springs into action and launches a general immune response consisting of a whole host of white blood cells, fever and biochemical complements to quickly eliminate an infection once it is detected.[50]

In contrast to this non-specific first line of defence, the body's adaptive immune system can remember and launch targeted attacks against specific pathogens. This adaptive response rests on specialised T-cells' ability to recognise specific molecules or molecular structures (antigens) produced by a pathogen and instruct the body to produce tailored antibodies and other immune cells to attack them.[51] [52]

The first antigen to be scientifically characterised was the toxin produced by *Cornyebacterium diphtheriae*, the bacterial cause of diphtheria. In 1888, future plague discoverer Alexandre Yersin and fellow microbiologist Émile Roux had discovered that this toxin was responsible for the lesions in diphtheria victims.[53] Further research soon revealed how tailored antibodies in the blood could bind to antigens and eliminate bacterial threats. In 1889, it was observed that *Pseudomonas* microbes were agglutinated (clumped together) by the serum of animals that had survived a previous pseudomonas infection.[54] Working on experimental treatments for diphtheria and tetanus in Germany, Emil von Behring and Shibasaburo Kitasato next reported in 1890 that injections of serum from animals exposed to tetanus and diphtheria could confer immunity to other animals. The observed immunity was conferred by antibodies (antitoxins), which could be isolated from the serum of an infected animal. In collaboration with their colleague, Paul Ehrlich, Kitasato and von Behring used purified diphtheria antibodies from infected animals to trial – allegedly on Christmas Eve 1891 – the first targeted treatment of diphtheria in a human. Their Nobel Prize-winning innovation not only laid the ground for a new era of serum therapy, but also opened the door for serum-based diagnostics.[53] [55] [56]

If specialised antibodies could combat an infection by agglutinating pathogens in the body, then similar antibody-antigen reactions might be useful to rapidly identify the presence of a pathogen in the laboratory or even at patients' bedsides. Between 1894 and 1896, bacteriologists in Berlin and Vienna began to develop serological diagnostics. In Berlin, Richard Pfeiffer reported that injecting live cultures of cholera and typhoid bacteria into guinea pigs, which had previously been exposed to live or heat-killed cultures of the same bacteria, led to the clumping and immobilisation of the live cultures. Clumping also occurred when live cultures were injected into non-immunised animals alongside the serum of previously exposed animals (Chapter 10). Significantly, live cultures of other bacteria species were not clumped. Other bacteriologists were eager to test Pfeiffer's reaction. In Vienna, bacteriologist Max von Gruber and his British collaborator Herbert Edward Durham accidentally discovered that clumping reactions could also be observed with the naked eye in test tubes. Gruber described the phenomenon as being due to specific agglutinins in the serum – thereby indirectly coining agglutination.[57] [58]

Both the Berlin and Viennese teams recognised the diagnostic value of these reactions. The fact that the serum of a typhoid survivor would agglutinate S. Typhi and not other organisms promised to speed up traditional confirmation, which consisted of lengthy culture-based and biochemical tests. In Vienna, Gruber began to study whether human sera could be used to confirm a specific infection in patients. In accordance with contemporary thinking, he concentrated on using supposedly more potent sera from convalescents, who had already achieved immunity.[17] This, however, meant that confirmation of an infection was retrospective.

It was left to French physician Georges Fernand Isidore Widal to first apply the principle of diagnostic agglutination reactions to an active infection. Born into a medical family near Algiers in 1862, Widal had trained in Paris under Roux and Metchnikoff, and started his research career in microbiology around 1886. In collaboration with fellow bacteriologist André Chantemesse, he initially studied streptococcal infections, bacterial virulence and typhoid immunisation and agglutination.[17] [57] His experience as a physician made Widal quickly realise the potential of using German and Austrian reports on selective agglutination to diagnose ongoing typhoid infections. Working with patients in Paris, Widal was able to show that the sera of still-febrile patients were already capable of agglutinating pure S. Typhi cultures. On 26 June 1896, Widal therefore proposed a new form of 'sero-diagnostics' as rapid point-of-care tests for infections at the conference of the Medical Society of the Paris Hospitals.* Rather than engage in arduous culturing of S. Typhi, he described adding:

---

* Working in parallel in Vienna under Gruber, Albert Sidney Grünbaum (later Leyton) developed a nearly identical rapid test that was slightly easier to use.

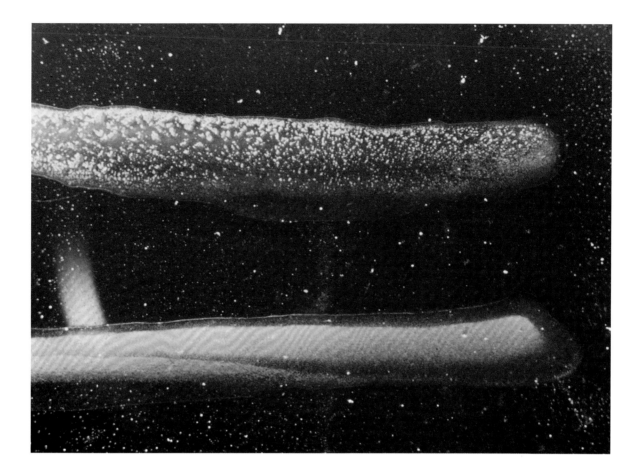

... a drop of serum or even a drop of blood taken from the tip of the finger of the patient to ten drops of a young culture in bouillon of typhoid fever bacilli [on a dish], and to see almost immediately under the microscope the formation of 'heaps' or agglomerations of bacilli, which often allows an almost instantaneous diagnosis of typhoid fever to be made.[45]

Widal's concept of sero-diagnostics was hugely influential, and quickly triggered research on serological tests for other organisms. In the case of typhoid, the so-called Widal-Gruber or Widal indirect agglutination test was soon being sold around the world as a ready-to-use kit. However, it turned out to be less precise than Widal had hoped. Many clinicians soon complained about false negatives or false positives in areas where high typhoid prevalence or vaccination levels meant that many people already had antibodies in their blood.**[59] Despite the development of more reliable automated tests for multiple serological markers since the 1990s,[60] resource constraints mean that the comparatively cheap Widal test is still used as a point-of-care test for typhoid in some poorer areas of the world.[61]

Many agglutination tests use a standardised serum to identify microbial isolates. This image of a slide agglutination test shows the agglutination (clumping) of the upper culture of *Vibrio cholerae* by antibodies in a cholera-specific serum. The lower control culture is still smooth.

** In 1934, the co-discovery of the so-called Vi (virulence) antigen by Margaret Pitt and Arthur Felix led to the development of sero-diagnostics, which could identify asymptomatic carriers in populations with high exposure to typhoid. Whereas the serum of most typhoid patients no longer contains Vi-antibodies after an infection has passed, many carriers continue to produce Vi-antibodies and their serum agglutinates purified Vi-antigens.

'A handy apparatus for the performance of the Widal-Gruber test for typhoid fever without the use of a microscope' (Messrs Parke Davis & Co., 1904): Four small tubes contain a suspension of dead typhoid bacilli.

STEP ONE

A few drops of blood are received into a 'blood tube';

STEP TWO

the serum, which separates, is drawn up into a glass tube with a rubber bulb;

STEP THREE

varying quantities of serum are dropped into the three typhoid suspensions;

STEP FOUR

these tubes are corked, shaken and placed in a warm room.

RESULT

If a positive agglutination reaction results, flocculi appear in one or more of the tubes and form a distinct layer at the bottom. A fourth tube is used as a control.

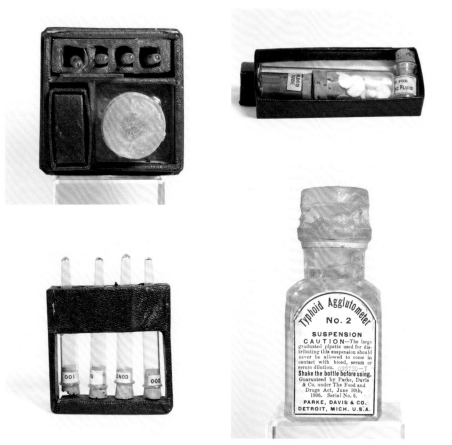

The nineteenth century thus saw a sea change in humans' relation with typhoid. At the beginning of the century, typhoid had been a more or less invisible part of the wider background noise of infectious fevers. As a result of international research, the years between 1829 and 1845 first saw typhoid fever become a distinct disease category that could be found in bodies due to its specific pathology and symptoms. Between the 1840s and 1870s, a mix of case tracing via Victorian shoe-leather epidemiology and new forms of data-gathering next turned typhoid into a disease whose spread could be traced, mapped and increasingly linked to contaminated water and food. Between 1880 and 1884, advances in microbiology transformed typhoid from an amorphous poison, exhalation or organism into a disease with a specific microbial cause (*S.* Typhi), which could be seen under the microscope, isolated from patients and the environment and manipulated on petri dishes. Finally, 1896 saw the development of a new form of sero-diagnostics that combined microbiological knowledge and immunological concepts of antigen/antibody reactions to identify *S.* Typhi in the blood. None of these innovations changed medical practice overnight, many blurred with pre-existing ways of making sense of disease and all took decades to be accepted as established dogma. However, taken together, these 67 years of ongoing research created the modern definition of typhoid that is still with us today.

3

Being able to see a problem is not to agree on one and the same solution. This is particularly true for public health. Since around 1900, microbiologists, engineers and public health experts have highlighted the decline of typhoid in richer European and American settings as proof of a 'great sanitary awakening'.[62] In Part Two, we saw that the nineteenth century had indeed led to fundamental shifts in the way typhoid was 'seen'. However, as Part Three will show, resulting public health gains occurred unevenly, were accompanied by strife and were by no means linear or irreversible. The complex political, cultural and environmental contexts in which medical, sanitary and hygiene interventions were trialled and implemented meant that following the science was never straightforward – especially since the voice of science itself was polyphone and constantly changing. This was particularly obvious in the case of the ethical dilemma resulting from the discovery that some typhoid survivors could shed S. Typhi years after seemingly recovering from an infection. Ultimately, controlling typhoid in wealthy cities like Oxford and New York or on battlefields in South Africa depended on having the 'right' science for the 'right' context, as well as the willingness and resources to implement this science.

OPPOSITE
A Boer War army medical officer standing in front of a tent with victims of enteric fever (see p.62).

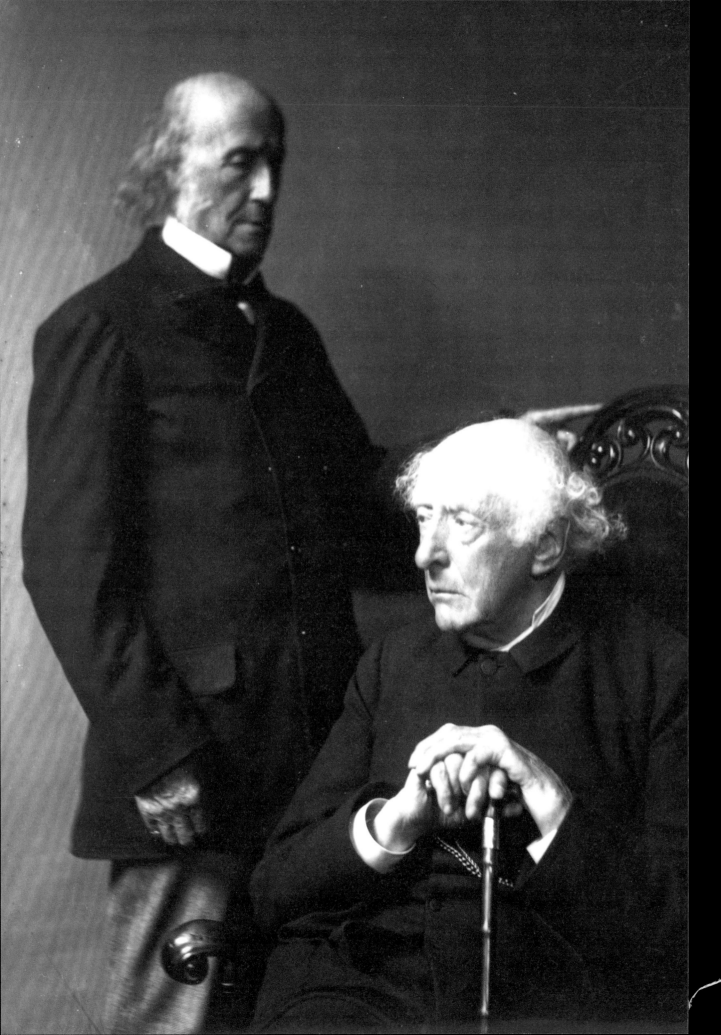

CHAPTER SEVEN

Sanitation in Wonderland

There can be no doubt that at the present moment Oxford is not a safe place of residence, owing to the imperfect condition of its drainage and impure water supply.

THE LANCET, 1875[63]

ACCESS to safe and affordable drinking water, as well as effective disposal of human excrement, is crucial in breaking the transmission chains of S. Typhi and other enteric pathogens.[64] However, providing both services to larger populations is not easy. The clean water coming out of our taps and – relatively – clean water in many of our rivers depends on significant and regular investment in sophisticated infrastructure. In rich areas of the globe, large parts of this infrastructure emerged in the late nineteenth century and continue to quietly do their work beneath our feet. The struggles surrounding their creation are often forgotten.

The following case study of evolving water infrastructures in the British city of Oxford between the 1860s and 1880s, when Lewis Carroll (Christ Church mathematician Charles Dodgson) was writing the *Alice in Wonderland* books, takes us to the heart of these sanitary conflicts. Like many other cities in flood-prone areas, Oxford has always struggled with its hydrological environment. The city lies in a narrow valley underlain by centuries of fertile alluvial deposits from its two rivers, the Isis (Thames) and the Cherwell. Its low-lying location at the heart of these two river systems not only gave the city its name – Oxnaford, Anglo-Saxon for 'ford of oxen' – but also caused many headaches about how to deal simultaneously with an excess of flood water and a lack of clean drinking water. While the original walled city was built on a spit of higher-lying gravel, Oxford's subsequent growth meant that an increasing number of buildings were built on the loose sediment of its flood-prone alluvial plains.[65]

Between the seventeenth and twentieth centuries, severe floods occurred regularly. In 1852, major flooding interrupted railway connections to London, flooded low-lying areas of the city and killed at least three inhabitants. Additional major floods occurred in 1892, 1903, 1947, 1954, 1959, 1979, 1998, 2007 and 2014.* For much of the Victorian era, ensuring that rainfall and sewage from medieval surface drains was rapidly transported away proved challenging even in times without major flooding. Guaranteeing access to drinkable water was equally difficult. With the city's weather becoming wetter, and with population levels increasing, sewage

OPPOSITE
A photograph (collodion lantern slide) of Henry Acland and Henry Liddell taken by Sarah Angelina Acland, 1898.

* Oxford's flood events have also been immortalised in children's fiction; see, for example, the major flood Malcolm Polstead experiences in *La Belle Sauvage*, the first part of Philip Pullman's *Book of Dust* trilogy.

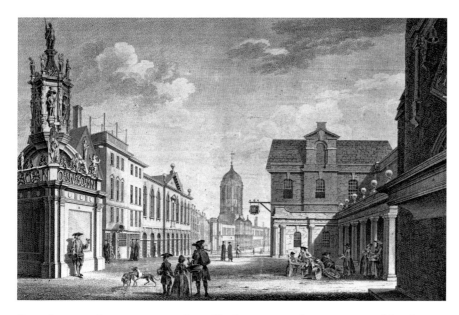

Conduit building at Carfax, 1775. Carfax Conduit supplied Oxford with fresh water between 1610 and 1869. The elaborate conduit building at Carfax consisted of an upper cistern, which supplied the university, and a lower, fed by the overflow, for the city. The building was replaced with a smaller cistern in 1797.

from drains and a growing number of leaking cesspools contaminated local rivers and the many shallow wells on which town inhabitants relied.[65]–[68]

Famed for its 'dreaming spires', the foundations of Oxford's many colleges and university buildings were in fact sunk into ground saturated with human faeces. Local residents were well aware of these problems. During 1851 hearings on the state of the city's sanitation, lower-lying parts of Oxford were described as a 'swamp converted into a cesspool'.[69] In many of the poorer low-lying areas of the city, such as Jericho, St Ebbes, St Clements and St Thomas, the growing density of cesspools had led to a saturation of entire areas with human effluent. One street had 14 cesspools in a space of about 25 yards square: 'The ground here is wholly a mass of corruption, arising from these cesspools; there is no chance of getting the matter away.'[69]

With wells and cesspools within a few feet of each other,[69] and residents defecating into the same hydrological environment they were drawing water from, rowing on and bathing in, the conditions were perfect for the circulation of typhoid. Things were made worse by the fact that since the seventeenth century, the city's waterworks had been drawing water downstream from 'nearly all the sewers'.[70] Perhaps fortunately, the high price of this dubious piped water meant that it remained out of reach for the vast majority of the city's inhabitants. In 1848, only 3.56% of dwellings had piped water.[71] According to the Health of Towns Association, municipal water supply was 'intermittent and very deficient'.[70] Despite upgrades in 1849 and 1850, only 340 premises (c.4,585 houses officially listed) were connected to the town supply, as well as 19 colleges, the University Printing Office and municipal buildings such as the County and City Gaols.[69]

The Oxford waterworks below the city's sewage outlets at Folly Bridge, 1825.

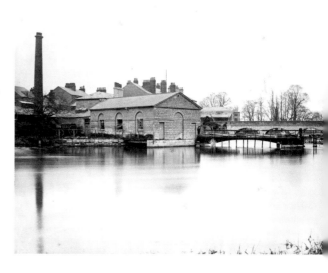

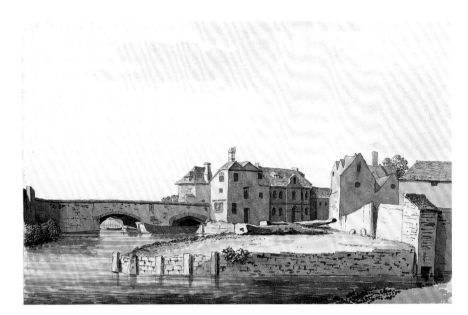

S.H. Grimm, view in ink of the junction between the rivers Pactolus and Isis, c.1777–81.

Safer water was only available to elites. Between 1617 and 1869, Carfax Conduit supplied university colleges and a small number of private homes. Springwater from surrounding hills was gathered in a cistern and piped into Oxford via lead pipes, and elm-encased pipes were used to cross over the Thames. An elaborate Conduit building gathered and distributed the water to recipients across Oxford.[71]

Although city authorities faced regular complaints about stench, sewage-contaminated watercourses and overflowing cesspools, it was not until the mid-nineteenth century that they launched concerted attempts to improve the situation.

Key to this move was a combination of scientific and political pressure, damaging scandals, cheap government credit and an alliance of university and municipal elites. The former group included lexicographer Henry Liddell, Dean of Christ Church and father of Alice Liddell (aka Alice in Wonderland), and his friend, the physician and alleged inspiration for the White Rabbit,[78] Henry Acland.

The two Henrys were deeply committed to sanitary reform. Liddell had gained a reputation for obsessing about drainage while heading Westminster School of Boys during the 1830s – where his wife, Lorina, had nearly died of typhoid. Although he probably thought of typhoid as a miasmatic 'air-borne' disease (Chapter 4), Liddell spent his first years as Dean of Christ Church trying to protect his family and students by pushing for improvements of the college's sanitary arrangements. This included improving water supplies, draining stagnant water and

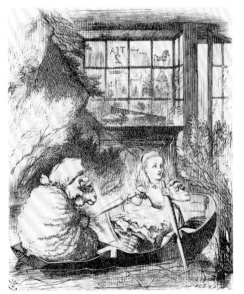

J. Tenniel, Alice and the White Queen – transformed into a talking sheep – travelling across a stream by rowboat, 1871.

working with city authorities to brick up Trill Mill Stream in 1863.[72] Also referred to by students as Pactolus, the gold-strewn river of myth, this foul-smelling sewer ran along Christ Church's borders before emptying into the Thames. It may also have been an inspiration for Alice's subterranean ride with the sheep, which featured in Lewis Carroll's *Through the Looking-Glass* in 1871.

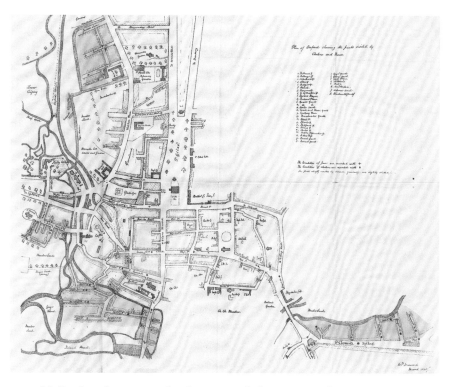

'Plan of Oxford Shewing the Parts Visited by Cholera and Fever', from W.R. Ormerod's *On the sanatory condition of Oxford*, 1848.[75]

Liddell's friend, Henry Acland, was similarly committed to sanitary reform. When cholera hit Oxford in 1849 and 1854,** Acland worked as a physician at the Radcliffe Infirmary. Having focused on treating patients in 1849, he tried to contain the 1854 outbreak as a consulting physician to Oxford's Board of Health. Under Acland's direction, authorities reacted to concerns that transferring cholera victims to local hospitals would meet with popular resistance by setting up a system of nursing people at home, distributing food and medicine, and designating a 'field of observation' to receive poor patients and monitor family contacts.[73] [74] Acland also trialled environmental interventions. During the previous cholera outbreak, the local county gaol had suffered higher fatalities than either the city prison or the workhouse. After hearing about rising cholera cases in the gaol, Acland found that water was taken from an often stagnant pool that also received the gaol's sewage. He successfully convinced the gaol's governor to disconnect this supply, and no further fatalities occurred.[73]

The cholera waves prompted Acland and his medical colleagues to campaign for sanitary reform. Using the familiar Victorian mix of shoe-leather epidemiology and statistics (see Part Two), they conducted extensive studies on how cholera and other 'fevers' spread through Oxford. Classism, uncertainties about the causes of disease, and their memories of difficult dealings with local politicians influenced both their investigations and findings.

Published between 1848 and 1856, reports by Acland and the Oxford surgeons William Ormerod, Thomas Allen and William Greenhill all emphasised the higher incidence of cholera and other 'fevers' in poorer, low-lying and over-crowded

** An earlier outbreak had already occurred in 1832.

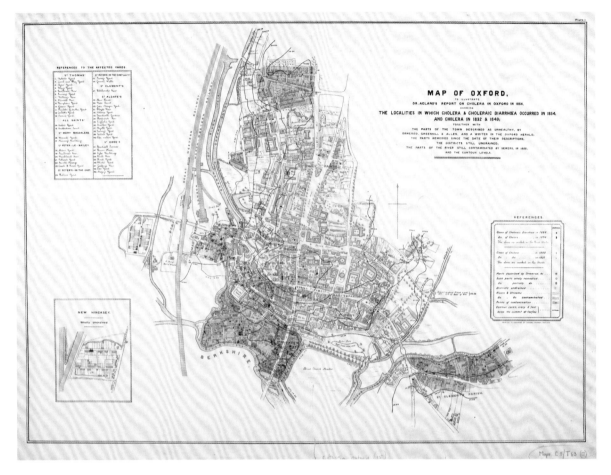

Henry Acland's map of cholera in Oxford, 1854.[73]

parishes with poor drainage and ventilation. In addition to drawing on national and local mortality and morbidity statistics, Ormerod and Acland described visiting filthy lower-class slum dwellings where contagion and immorality had been rife. They also printed maps to illustrate their findings.[73] [75] [76] Ormerod's hand-drawn 1848 map was basic in its depiction of localities of 'fever' and cholera cases, and shaded areas of high prevalence, which were characterised by bad drainage and proximity to putrefying filth. By contrast, Acland's 1856 map looks far more contemporary with its John Snow-style dotmap (Chapter 4) of historical and current cholera cases and detailed attention to sewage outlets and contaminated water-courses. However, a closer look at the altitude lines running across Oxford also reveals ongoing uncertainties about the ways diseases like cholera spread.

In his accompanying report, Acland drew on his own county gaol intervention and recent publications by John Snow to underline 'the immediate connection between the Water and the existence of the Disease'.[73] However, he was unconvinced that waterborne transmission could explain all observed cases of cholera, such as that of a farm labourer who had died suddenly, miles away from any contaminated water. Additional factors seemed to be at play. Like other contemporaries (Chapter 4), Acland painstakingly compiled data on potentially contributing environmental, social and meteorological conditions. His final report featured four pages on Oxford's water and drainage, and over 16 on temperature, ozone, rain, wind and cloud coverage. Fusing contagionist and anti-contagionist theories, Acland argued that cholera could arise without any connection to previous cases and then spread in a contagious manner via foul water and air.[23] [33] [73]

Significantly, Acland argued that inhabitants of Oxford were 'now in a position to calculate their safety in a future Epidemic, and to form an estimate of the propriety of adopting such preventive sanitary measures as experience and science suggest'.[73] Encoded in this recommendation was a broad programme of sanitary and social reform, as well as a challenge to local politicians in the area of public health. According to Acland and his allies, medical experts should not only guide epidemic emergency responses, but should also obtain political influence when it came to upgrading Oxford's sanitary infra-structure and health arrangements. Prevention entailed targeting both the factors contributing to the spontaneous emergence of 'fevers' such as cholera as well as subsequent transmission routes. In concrete terms, this meant rapidly removing contagious agents by improving ventilation and drainage throughout Oxford, disinfecting discharges from patients and improving the living conditions and moral state of the city's poorest inhabitants. Because disease in lower and undrained parishes also endangered inhabitants of higher and wealthier parts of Oxford, preventive action was in the self-interest of the entire city.[73] Effective prevention would entail implementing provisions of the 1848 Public Health Act and coordinating action by municipal officials and the powerful university.

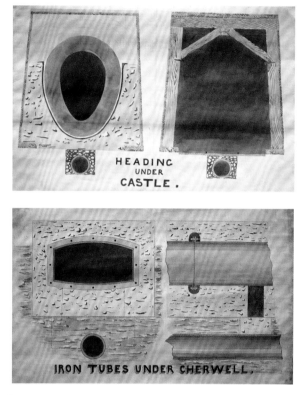

Drawings showing details of Oxford's main drainage plan (c.1870).

Not everyone agreed. Similar to the national controversies about the sanitary ideas of Chadwick and Farr (Part Two), local critics attacked Oxford sanitarians' calls for reform. Some doubted that stagnant water was dangerous, while others believed that flooding was a blessing rather than a curse, because it washed filth away. Resulting criticism also revealed distrust of the national government and deep rifts between the university and leading townspeople. While the university's commissioners supported proposals for sanitary reform, many town representatives opposed sanitarians' expensive plans, for which the university refused to pay, and which would have entailed a loss of local autonomy.[66] [77] [78]

The resulting political stalemate was characterised by acrimonious exchanges in newspapers and council meetings, as well as numerous reports on the state of Oxford's public health and sanitation. Between 1851 and 1870, the city saw no fewer than nine different proposals to overhaul Oxford's public health and sanitation. Although their proposals varied, the reports revealed an emerging alliance between campaigning university physicians such as Acland, who was promoted to Regius Professor of Medicine in 1858, and members of the young and confident discipline of civil engineers. Both sides gravitated towards radical hydrological intervention. Together with his friend Dean Liddell, Acland supported an ultimately fruitless campaign to dredge the Thames, redirect the Cherwell and cut through a medieval lock at Iffley to increase water flow, reduce flood risks and drain Thames tributaries. Liddell and Acland also supported plans to separate man-made and natural water flows by pumping Oxford's sewage through miles of pipes and bricked sewers to a municipal sewage farm. Far less attention was devoted to how sanitary interventions could be coupled with improving the living conditions of the poorest citizens, who suffered the highest disease burdens.[78]–[81]

The focus on removing sewage and odiferous filth also led to a relative neglect of the city's water supply. Although they stopped pumping Thames water from below sewage outlets in 1853, Oxford authorities ignored advice for new waterworks to be situated upstream of the city, and instead acquired cheap spring-fed gravel pits that had been excavated by the Great Western Railway. The new 'lake' was situated close to the sewage-contaminated Thames and the cesspits of the expanding Hinksey neighbourhood. It was also occasionally topped up with Thames water and at risk of contamination during floods. Despite improved pumping and simple gravel and sand filtration, the high cost and varying quality of municipal water made the majority of Oxford's inhabitants continue to favour local wells or even river water.[78]

Wonderland's 20-year sanitary stalemate was only broken as a result of embarrassment about typhoid outbreaks – particularly among university elites – cheap national credit and a new 'town and gown' alliance for sanitary investment. By 1870, there was growing consensus about the role that contaminated water played in spreading typhoid. Meanwhile, Chief Medical Officer (CMO) John Simon's labelling of typhoid as a preventable 'filth' disease placed increasing pressure on local authorities to upgrade water infrastructures (Part Two).[3] Oxford did not cut a good figure in national comparisons. In 1871, CMO Simon publicly criticised the poor state of Oxford's public health and sanitary arrangements.[66] From 1866 onwards, town authorities also faced legal action under the new Thames Navigation Act and from the unified Thames Conservancy to stop draining and pumping sewage into the Thames.[82]

Pressure to change course was also mounting on university authorities. With the avid sanitarian Henry Liddell heading the university as Vice-Chancellor between 1870 and 1874, university authorities were keenly aware of the reputational damage that typhoid outbreaks could cause. Reports on high local typhoid incidence were particularly concerning since a growing number of students no longer lived on university-owned premises. In a break with tradition, Oxford

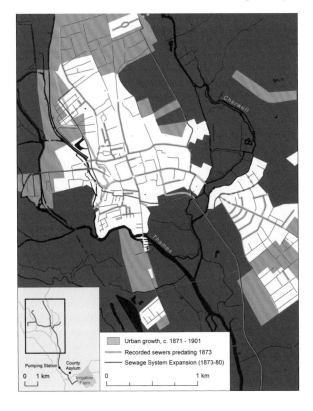

The expansion of Oxford and its sewage system, 1871–1901.

Urban growth, c. 1871 - 1901
Recorded sewers predating 1873
Sewage System Expansion (1873-80)

Pumping Station   County Asylum
0   1 km   Irrigation Farm

0   1 km

University had permitted poorer students to live in non-college lodging from the 1860s onwards. While typhoid outbreaks also occurred inside college walls, some of the new lodging houses were situated in poorer neighbourhoods, which were particularly prone to the disease. In 1874, the death of three of four undergraduates who had contracted typhoid in Oxford lodging houses made national news[78] – especially since one of them was the son of Liberal MP Samuel Laing.[83] Resulting parliamentary questions and a sanitary commission by *The Lancet* threatened Oxford's reputation as an educational destination for Britain's upper classes by describing the local water supply as 'disgraceful', the condition of low-lying suburbs as 'deplorable',[84] and by stating that 'Oxford is not a safe place of residence'.[63] [85] Adding insult to injury, it was also rumoured that Prince Leopold, Queen Victoria's youngest son, had contracted typhoid while living in Oxford and studying at Christ Church.[86]

With pressure mounting, municipal and university authorities agreed on a programme of investment. Aided by cheap national and local credit,[87] the first area of concern to be tackled by the new 'town and gown' alliance was Oxford's sewage. In 1870, the city's engineer, William Henry White, was tasked with drawing up an ambitious sewerage plan for the entire city that was based on a proposal by sanitary engineer Baldwin Latham and projected to cost £40,000.[88] [78] Following endorsements by university experts and municipal and district officials in 1871, construction commenced in 1872. The new system consisted of a 33-mile London-inspired mix of bricked and egg-shaped clay sewers, as well as cast-iron pipes. Construction was accompanied by the demolition or repurposing of older wastewater systems. By 1880, most existing cesspits and privies had been demolished or filled in, medieval sewers were converted to drain only rainwater, and new flushing water closets were connected to White's sewers. These sewers and pipes then transported the city's sewage across the rivers Thames and Cherwell to Sandford, where it was screened and pumped up to a 370-acre sewage farm at Littlemore – close to the so-called County Lunatic Asylum. On the farm, the sewage was passed into earth-banked lagoons to allow heavier solids to settle, while liquid overflowed onto adjacent land, where it then percolated through the soil and aerated. When not receiving sewage, land on the farm was used to produce rye grass, crop and osier, as well as for cattle grazing.[65] [78] [89] [90] In preparation for the influx of sewage construction workers, local authorities also decided to hire Oxford's first permanent Medical Officer of Health to control disease and advise on sanitary measures going forward.[91]

Construction was accompanied by further strife. There were disagreements about the placement of ventilation shafts, the frequency of sewer flushing, the partial choice of bricked rather than glazed earthenware sewers, the safety of food produced on the new sewage farm and potential pollution and health hazards for the local asylum.[92]–[97] The decision to route the main sewers over the Cherwell, just below Magdalen Bridge – one of the city's most popular tourist spots – and temporarily redirect all sewers towards an old outfall next to Magdalen College led to complaints about 'abominable stench' and sewage backflow.[98] Meanwhile, local newspapers and national journals such as *The Lancet* printed debates about the relative merits of different closet systems, the water- or airborne transmission of typhoid and cholera, and the alleged danger of

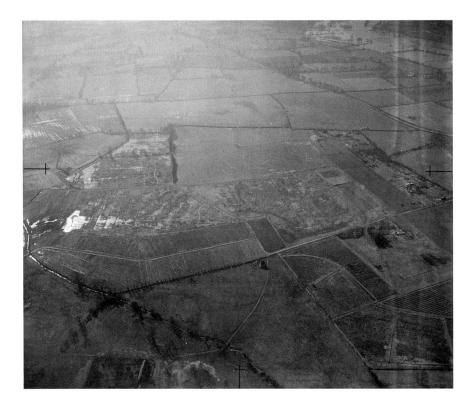

sewer gases escaping through water closets – which Acland believed had infected Prince Leopold with typhoid.[99]–[103] † There were also tensions between university and town officials when it came to mandating the improvement of student lodging houses not owned by the university.[104]

Sanitarians' focus on removing sewage meant that sustained efforts to improve Oxford's water supply only began during the second half of the 1870s. In 1875, sharp criticism by a *Lancet* Commission prompted local authorities to promise to prevent the sewage contamination of the municipal water supply.[105] Between 1878 and 1885, Oxford used funds from the British Waterworks Bill to install pump-fed, slow-sand filtration beds for water from its Hinksey Lake reservoir. Filtered water was pumped to a covered freshwater reservoir on Headington Hill, from where it fed the growing city with gravity pressure. The new system started work in June 1885. To protect the purity of its water, Oxford also invested in a new supplemental water intake above the city at Kings Weir and disconnected its reservoir from Hogs Weir stream, which had been used to top up supplies with unfiltered Thames water. To ensure maximum uptake – and reduce use of contaminated wells – officials followed the example of other cities and adopted a rate-financed system, which forced all households to use municipal water but made contributions in the form of a tax dependent on property value and income. By 1886, the majority of Oxford's houses were connected to an affordable, financially sustainable and increasingly safe water supply and sewage

---

† As personal physician to Leopold, and 'knowing only too well the susceptibility of the members of the Royal Family to typhoid', Acland had allegedly campaigned against connecting Leopold's residence at Wykeham House to Oxford's sewer system.[74]

disposal system.[78] [106] Commenting on the at times glacial pace of progress, *The Lancet* highlighted the role of public pressure in driving action:

> Indeed, by this time the city authorities at Oxford must feel that it is hard to kick against the pricks of public opinion. It was public opinion that forced them to adopt their present system of sewerage. It was public opinion, after a long struggle, which made them abandon their old reservoir at Hincksey [sic] ... and now the lodgings of the undergraduates are to be made healthy in spite of them.[107]

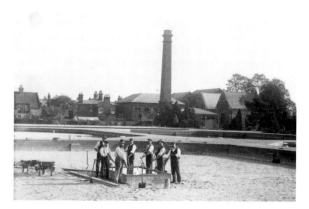

Workmen washing sand-filter beds at the Hinksey waterworks, 1914.

The combination of safe water provision and effective sewage disposal had an impressive impact on local typhoid incidence. Although contemporary data is imprecise and patchy, it is possible to infer broader shifts of disease prevalence. Reporting by Oxford's Medical Officer of Health between 1870 and 1901 indicates a sharp dip of typhoid prevalence following the completion of the first phase of sewage construction and establishment of clean water supplies. Because both systems had been designed for maximum access, effects were not limited to richer inhabitants but were felt throughout the city. Further expansions of sewerage and water provision occurred in 1884 and 1920, and a new upstream waterworks at Swinford became operational in 1934. In a creative reuse of civic infrastructure, the filtration beds of the old waterworks at Hinksey were repurposed as an open-air swimming pool.[65] [78]

The introduction of chlorination in 1930 added an extra layer of protection for Oxford's water supply. Some typhoid researchers, such as William Budd, had advocated using solutions of chloride of zinc to disinfect the discharges of patients since the 1850s.[29] The gradual rise of germ theory added weight to these demands. In the German city of Hamburg, a notorious 1892 outbreak of cholera prompted officials to use large amounts of chloride of lime to clean houses, disinfect sewage and waterways, and temporarily chlorinate municipal wastewater in response to a subsequent typhoid outbreak.[108] [109] ‡ Parallel disinfection attempts with ozone were carried out in France. In 1896, Pola on the Adriatic coast had its water treated with chlorine. In Britain, Maidstone became the first city to treat its entire water supply, using ten tons of chloride of lime during a large-scale typhoid outbreak in 1897, which also saw the first large-scale trial of first-generation typhoid vaccines (Chapter 10).[108] [110] Eight years later, the English city of Lincoln followed the lead of Middelkerke and Ostende in Belgium in adopting permanent chlorination.[111] In the US, sanitary engineer John L. Leal subsequently constructed the first full-scale modern chlorination plant, which used a gravity feed of dilute solutions of chloride of lime to treat water from Jersey City's Boonton Reservoir – a technique that was later substituted with chlorine gas.[112]

‡ The episode also allowed microbiologist Koch to prove the comparative efficacy of sand-filtration systems in protecting citizens of Altona, downstream of Hamburg, from a similarly severe outbreak.

But were any of these developments inevitable? In Oxford, local authorities took great pride in a steady reduction of typhoid incidence – especially when a *Lancet* comparison between Oxford and Cambridge praised Oxford's drainage initiatives.[113]–[115] In 1887, Oxford's Medical Officer of Health confidently predicted that 'this formidable disease ought to become a thing of the past'.[116] While his prediction proved correct for Oxford, it would be wrong to think of the described history as an example of scientific knowledge leading to inexorable progress. Instead of a great sanitary awakening, the evolution of Oxford's sanitation was more resemblant of a fitful slumber.

Early disease statistics and maps were designed to reify authors' multi-causal interpretations of disease transmission during a time of unstable consensus on typhoid's aetiology. Oxfordshire's Medical Officer of Health, Gilbert Child, doubted the validity and usefulness of local, regional and national disease statistics as late as 1875 – prompting fierce attacks by *The Lancet*.[117] Henry Acland, whose son, Herbert, died of typhoid while working as a coffee planter in Sri Lanka in 1877,[74] eventually converted to germ theory and discussed monitoring Thames water for typhoid 'bacilli' with Joseph Lister in 1891.[118] However, he continued to warn about airborne transmission up to the mid 1870s.[99] Similarly, the city of Oxford's long-standing Medical Officer of Health, Alfred Winkfield, continued to follow older models of disease transmission via smell and poisons until shortly before his retirement in 1901.[66] Proposed sanitary solutions also mirrored the interests of distinct groups. While engineers and physicians favoured radical hydrological schemes, city officials gravitated towards less expensive interventions in a bid to maintain their independence from the national government, while university authorities favoured those they would not have to pay for. Tellingly, most of these elite reformers did not integrate their proposals for sanitary improvement with broader programmes of social support for Oxford's poorest. When they did come, sanitary interventions resulted not from grand master plans, but were trial-and-error compromises

Oxford enteric fever deaths in different areas of the city per 1,000 inhabitants between 1872 and 1901. The map highlights the higher disease burdens in the crowded low-lying parts of the city, and the significant improvement of the health of all parts of the city resulting from nineteenth-century sanitary upgrades.

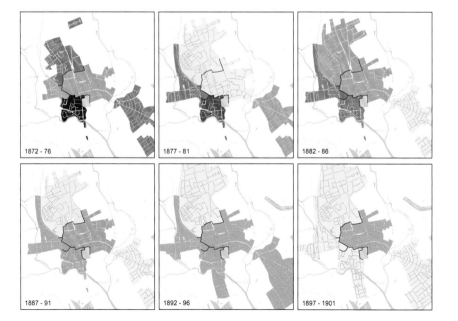

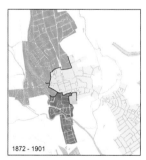

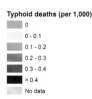

Typhoid deaths (per 1,000)

- 0
- 0 - 0.1
- 0.1 - 0.2
- 0.2 - 0.3
- 0.3 - 0.4
- > 0.4
- No data

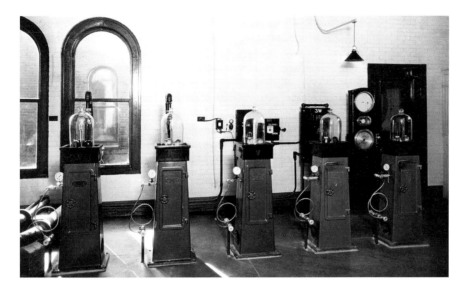

Chlorinator machines used inside the Minneapolis water filtration plant, 1917.

triggered by scandalous typhoid outbreaks, external pressure and cheap credit.

Seen from this perspective, the fact that Oxford's sanitary interventions managed to reduce typhoid incidence owed more to financial, geographic and environmental luck than to researchers' growing knowledge of the disease. An abundant supply of cleaner water was available just upstream of the city boundaries, and a viable disposal option was available in the form of the Littlemore sewage farm. Their choice of a sewage farm model and ability to finance miles of additional sewers to supply the farm is also testament to the ability of the city's well-connected elites to tailor water systems to the local environment.

Around the world, many areas do not have access to similar financial resources, clean water or sewage disposal options. In the US, cities including Chicago and San Francisco needed to develop different approaches, such as reversing the flows of rivers or building massive freshwater reservoirs to solve their unique sanitary challenges.[78] Meanwhile, civic engineers working in colonial contexts found that transplanting British sanitary designs into different hydrological and agricultural environments could lead to unintended consequences. In Dublin, pumping sewage into the Liffey estuary polluted shellfish banks with *S*. Typhi.[119] While sewage farms were hailed as a great success by their British and German promoters,[90] [120] the adoption of sewage irrigation in Paris and Santiago de Chile led to high rates of typhoid because of the production of leafy salad vegetables rather than the grass, cereal and meat that was produced in Oxford and Berlin.[120]–[122] § Many other localities simply did not have the financial and political resources to construct, maintain and guarantee widespread access to the water systems being pioneered in wealthy European and North American countries. To this day, one in four people have no access to safe drinking water, and nearly half of the world has no access to safe sanitation.[124]

§ The Oxford sewage farm was decommissioned in the 1950s. Sewage farms around Berlin were active until the 1980s and contaminated soils with metals, persistent organic compounds and pesticides.[89] [123]

CHAPTER EIGHT

Typhoid
on the table

The oysters transplanted from the coast of the county of
Wexford to the northern shores of Dublin Bay had, in recent
years, been much subject to disease, and had died in large
numbers ... Analyses of the sea-water at the oyster-beds ...
showed that [at low tide] the oysters were literally bathed
in sewage ... If typhoid could be transmitted through the
media of potable water and milk, was it not at least as likely
that oysters taken raw might ... also be the vehicle ...
of typhoid fever or other disease.

CHARLES A. CAMERON, 1880[125]

FOOD forms a second important mode of typhoid transmission. With water systems improving and typhoid rates declining from around 1900, European and North American authorities began to pay greater attention to how *S.* Typhi entered and spread via foodstuffs. Scientifically, resulting findings would pave the way for an increasingly complex understanding of how human, animal and environmental health were linked.[3] [4] From a public health perspective, they would also create new – often heavily moralised – expectations for hygienic behaviour at the level of businesses and of individuals.

At the level of the individual, the new bacteriological and epidemiological knowledge of typhoid transmission fused seamlessly with long-standing cultural equations of cleanliness and godliness. Gendered role models meant that females were often under particular social pressure to prevent themselves and family members from contracting a shameful 'filth-borne' disease. Responsibilities included scrupulously cleaning and airing houses, maintaining drains, combatting disease-carrying pests such as flies[126] and ensuring that food was stored and prepared in safe and hygienic ways. With bacteriological investigations highlighting how *S.* Typhi and other pathogens could spread via contaminated bodies, utensils and food, new aseptic thinking gradually made its way from the clinic to the kitchen.[127]

However, even the best hygiene practices were compromised if the food entering a household had already been contaminated during production. In the case of typhoid, three groups of foodstuffs emerged as particularly risky: raw milk, shellfish and leafy vegetables. In an age prior to widespread pasteurisation, faecal contamination of milk on farms or in dairies could lead to explosive community outbreaks. In the case of shellfish and leafy vegetables such as watercress, production and harvesting in estuaries, rivers and streams that carried sewage frequently led to *S.* Typhi contamination. All three industries would have to adapt their production methods in response to new bacteriological thinking.

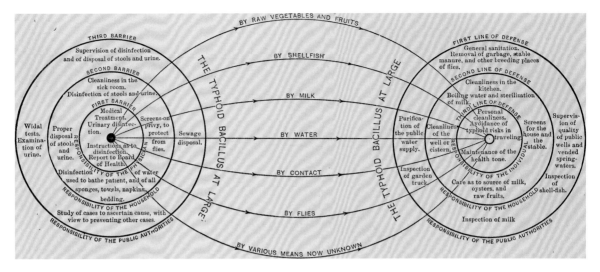

The diagram is labelled with the following text:

BY RAW VEGETABLES AND FRUITS

THIRD BARRIER
Supervision of disinfection and of disposal of stools and urine.

SECOND BARRIER
Cleanliness in the sick room.
Disinfection of stools and urine.

FIRST BARRIER
Medical Treatment.
Urinary disinfection.
Instructions as to disinfection.
Report to Board of Health.

Screens on privy, to protect from flies.

Sewage disposal.

Widal tests. Examination of urine.

Proper disposal of stools and urine.

RESPONSIBILITY OF THE PHYSICIAN

Disinfection of water used to bathe patient, and of all sponges, towels, napkins, bedding.

RESPONSIBILITY OF THE HOUSEHOLD

Study of cases to ascertain cause, with view to preventing other cases.

RESPONSIBILITY OF THE PUBLIC AUTHORITIES

THE TYPHOID BACILLUS AT LARGE

BY SHELLFISH
BY MILK
BY WATER
BY CONTACT
BY FLIES
BY VARIOUS MEANS NOW UNKNOWN

THE TYPHOID BACILLUS AT LARGE

FIRST LINE OF DEFENSE
General sanitation.
Removal of garbage, stable manure, and other breeding places of flies.

SECOND LINE OF DEFENSE
Cleanliness in the kitchen.
Boiling water and sterilization of milk.

THIRD LINE OF DEFENSE
Personal cleanliness.
Avoidance of typhoid risks in traveling.

Purification of the public water supply.

Cleanliness of the well or cistern.

Maintenance of the health tone.

Screens for the house and the stable.

Supervision of quality of public wells and vended spring-waters.

Inspection of garden truck.

RESPONSIBILITY OF THE INDIVIDUAL

Care as to source of milk, oysters, and raw fruits.

Inspection of shell-fish.

RESPONSIBILITY OF THE HOUSEHOLD

Inspection of milk

RESPONSIBILITY OF THE PUBLIC AUTHORITIES

Depiction of the known routes of typhoid transmission, 1908.

The shellfish trade was particularly impacted by changing understandings of typhoid transmission. Since the mid-nineteenth century, the increase of water-based sewage disposal systems had led to a significant rise of human effluent being washed through rivers and into coastal estuaries (see Chapter 7). However, the displaced sewage soon came back to haunt health officials. In 1880, Charles Cameron, the Medical Officer of Health in British-ruled Dublin, was one of the first to warn about sewage 'bathing' shellfish banks on the northern shore of Dublin Bay. With Oxford's Henry Acland in the audience, Cameron drew parallels to epidemiological investigations of water- and milkborne typhoid outbreaks, warning that sewage-tainted shellfish were contributing to typhoid in Dublin and spreading infection among poorer parts of the population, such as day labourers, petty clerks, small shopkeepers and hawkers.[4] [119]

While Cameron's warnings were initially disregarded by most experts, alarm increased in 1891 when Prince George (the future King George V) was said to have contracted typhoid after eating sewage-contaminated oysters in Dublin. The fact that yet another member of the royal family had come down with the disease caused widespread attention and prompted the shellfish trade to warn about the sewage contamination of other estuaries. Fears peaked after cholera returned to Western Europe around 1892 and epidemiological investigation linked some cases to the consumption of sewage-tainted shellfish. An 1894 investigation of a mass outbreak of typhoid at a fraternity supper in the US found similar evidence regarding typhoid.[4] [128]

The new findings cast a shadow over several popular shellfish species, such as cockles, periwinkles and mussels, but caused particular alarm about oysters, which – unlike today – were a popular working- and middle-class staple. In Britain, the mounting 'oyster scare' laid the ground for a new Oyster Bill, which proposed banning the removal of oysters from unsanitary beds, and regulating imports. The bill was eventually defeated, but it triggered sanitary

Raking watercress, River Lea, c.1930.

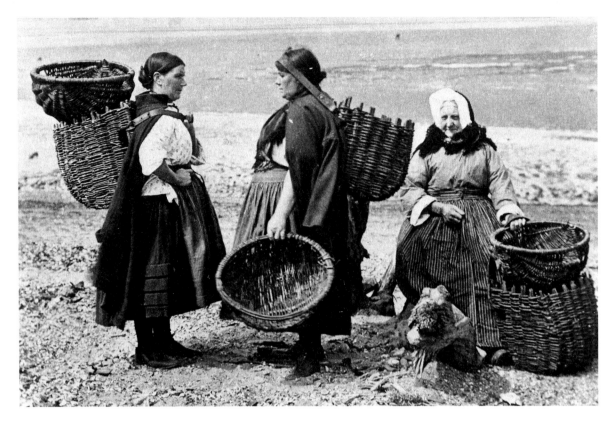

John J. Clarke, three cockle-pickers on an Irish beach, c.1890–1910.

guidelines for the production and subsequent purification of shellfish in clean water. It also prompted the increasingly influential discipline of bacteriology to develop tests for sewage contamination using proxy organisms such as E. coli (Klein's test).[4]

Typhoid scares also impacted the production of root and leafy vegetables – most notably, watercress. The popular aquatic member of the cabbage family was grown in streams, praised for its health-giving properties and often freshened up with untreated water prior to selling it. Contemporaries had begun to suspect, from the 1870s, that growing watercress in sewage-contaminated streams could pose health hazards. However, similar to oysters, it was only around 1900 that heightened fears of cholera and new bacteriology-informed investigations of urban typhoid outbreaks conclusively implicated sewage-contaminated watercress in the spread of S. Typhi.[129] [130]

Contamination risks were not limited to sewage exposure in streams, rivers and the ocean. During the interwar period, research revealed additional 'long cycle' hazards resulting from growing leafy and root vegetables in soil impregnated with untreated sewage. Researchers were able to isolate viable S. Typhi from vegetables such as radishes and lettuce produced on these soils for longer than it took to grow and harvest a plant. Although it was nearly impossible to disinfect fresh vegetables without boiling them, little formal regulation of growers or sewage farms seems to have followed. Instead, a gradual shift of production to less polluted – often non-urban – locations was driven by a mix of consumer demand and savvy rural producers capitalising on food safety concerns.[122] [129]–[132]

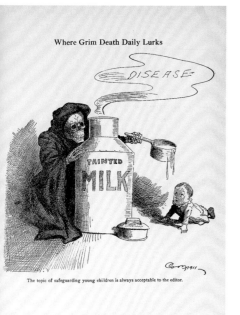

Where Grim Death Daily Lurks

DISEASE

TAINTED MILK

The topic of safeguarding young children is always acceptable to the editor.

Typhoid-tainted milk emerged as an even greater concern for public health authorities. As a highly prized form of nutrition for children, convalescents and the elderly, milk was consumed in large quantities by wealthier households and was subjected to increasingly stringent sanitary controls in the late nineteenth century.[133] Epidemiological investigations had started to link milk to the spread of typhoid and scarlet fever since the early 1870s. However, in the absence of agreement on typhoid's cause and mode of transmission (Chapter 4), public health interventions evolved unevenly. Although pasteurisation was developed during the 1860s, it was initially used to prevent spoilage of alcoholic beverages. In the case of milk, popular concepts of typhoid as a 'filth-borne' disease instead mixed with growing concerns about adulteration and led to a strong focus on cleanliness and quality assurance on farms and in dairies.[134] Concerns about filth also boosted attempts to remove commercial animal production from urban areas, introduce veterinary inspections at abattoirs and regulate food processing.[4] The overall impact of these filth-focused interventions on typhoid incidence was limited. While sanitary interventions could remove filth from animals and filthy animals from human cities, they offered only limited protection against the introduction and spread of microbial pathogens such as typhoid in food and milk.

The rise of germ theory increasingly challenged filth-based approaches to food safety. Bacteriologists confirmed chains of foodborne transmission that had long been suspected by epidemiologists and managed to culture the same pathogens from humans, foodstuffs and animals. Streptococci (scarlet fever) were isolated from humans, animals and milk around 1886,[135] and S. Typhi was isolated from milk in 1905.[136] However, it was the association of tuberculosis with milk that caused by far the greatest scare. Links between tuberculosis in humans and cows had long been suspected. During the 1880s and 1890s, bacteriological and epidemiological investigations confirmed that meat and milk from diseased cows could spread the disease to other species, but that Mycobacterium bovis, the cause of bovine tuberculosis, was distinct from Mycobacterium tuberculosis, which had been isolated in 1882.[137]–[139]

TB concerns triggered an explosion of interest in bacteriologically pure milk. Consumer concerns merged with Progressive Era campaigns to reduce child mortality. In the eyes of many, pasteurisation became the most promising way to guarantee pure and safe milk. The first commercial pasteurisation process for milk had been developed in Germany in 1882, and heat treatment for bottled milk, which was becoming an increasingly popular food for infants, was developed in 1886. By heating milk to below 100°C, pasteurisation not only killed dangerous pathogens such as S. Typhi or M. bovis, but also increased shelf life. However, different forms of pasteurisation could alter the taste of milk, and not every early process was effective in eliminating pathogens.[140]

There was also more fundamental opposition to the technology. Some feared that prolonged heating of milk denatured and devitalised a nutritious and health-giving natural product. Others preferred raw milk precisely because of its freshness. Robert Koch caused further controversy around 1901 by claiming that bovine tuberculosis posed little threat to humans. Resulting controversies led to divergent hygiene regimes. After initially remaining on the fence, a growing number of larger dairies began to invest in pasteurisation to gain a competitive advantage. Meanwhile, countries such as Germany and Denmark, as well as some larger US cities, made pasteurisation compulsory. By contrast, British authorities shied away from intervening in the milk market, and the majority of British milk outside of London remained raw until the post-war period.[133] [140] [141]

All of this must have been deeply confusing for turn-of-the-century consumers. In contrast to later stories of a revolutionary age of bacteriological reform, people's day-to-day reality was often one of uncertainty and anxiety.[127] [142] [143] Having been trained to think in terms of filth, poisons and miasma, consumers were now being exhorted to be wary of produce that could look, taste and smell completely innocuous – despite it teeming with invisible pathogens. What is more, many of the particularly risky products, such as oysters, watercress and milk, were those whose freshness was heralded as health-giving. At the same time, expert advice and regulations remained riven by contradiction, and producer organisations often disagreed with health warnings that threatened long-standing production practices.[4] Contemporary bacteriologists' difficulty in isolating pathogens such as *S.* Typhi from food and the environment also meant that they were often unable to provide proof of foodborne transmission during or following outbreaks. This led to uncertainty about which form of food production, and whose authority, to trust. Writing to *The Times* in 1896, 'A Layman' expressed concern about the soundness of bacteriologists' warnings about typhoid tainted oysters:

> Cannot some other expert give us a little comfort about the typhoid germ? Can it be true that the bacillus of typhoid is not to be distinguished from a crowd of similar but innocuous bacteria? I have heard it say – by one having authority – that no single one of the very few bacteria which can with certainty be associated with a definite disease has ever, with certainty, been found in water (not to say oysters). It would be a great comfort to us outsiders to believe this. Would somebody tell us if we may.[144]

The decades after 1900 saw a significant increase in the proportion of milk that was pasteurised. This leaflet, c.1930–37, informs consumers how milk produced by the Co-operative Union is made safe by pasteurisation.

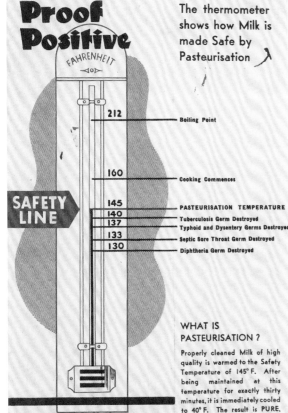

CHAPTER NINE

Typhoid and Mary

> Previously, one assumed – as I also did originally – that ...
> the typhoid bacillus was ... able to live a saprophyte life
> [on dead or decaying matter] ... When one has the
> opportunity to analyse the small typhoid epidemics in rural
> areas ... one finds regularly that individual cases are
> connected to each other. ... Our experiment ... proves firstly
> that an offensive campaign against typhoid ... is possible and
> secondly proves that there is indeed no other source of
> typhoid infection than the human.
>
> ROBERT KOCH, 1902[145]

The growing acceptance of germ theory around 1900 also opened new ways of thinking about disease reservoirs. Victorian campaigns against 'filth-borne' typhoid had led to a substantial reduction of typhoid incidence in many European and North American territories. However, important questions remained about where *S.* Typhi resided between outbreaks. Although epidemiological case-mapping and early bacteriology had identified the main pathways of *S.* Typhi transmission, researchers struggled to explain why even the most hygienic communities continued to experience low endemic levels of typhoid. Looking to other diseases for answers, some speculated that typhoid must spread to humans as a zoonotic infection from animals, persist in spore form in the environment or that underreporting of active cases in humans obscured ongoing chains of transmission. Linking epidemiology and bacteriology provided a more disturbing scenario: could seemingly healthy humans be harbouring and spreading the bacteria?

The concept of so-called asymptomatic carriage ran counter to early bacteriological theories according to which known pathogens were necessary causes of clinical disease but was increasingly supported by data from closely monitored military and colonial populations. During the Spanish-American War of 1898, the US Army had made substantial use of new Widal tests and culture-based screening of soldiers to prevent typhoid (Chapters 5 and 6). When analysing resulting data, US military physician Walter Reed concluded that outbreaks in army camps must have originated from 'healthy' asymptomatic carriers, who shed *S.* Typhi in their faeces and urine.[146] [147] * In Germany, Robert Koch had similar suspicions. While working

---

* Other US-based researchers, such as Harvey Cushing, were also uncovering evidence of healthy carriers.[17]

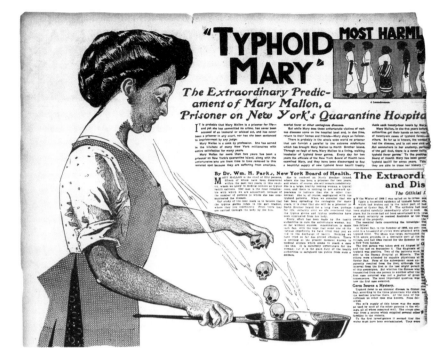

Mary Mallon was branded 'Typhoid Mary' in the press, 1909.

in the African and Asian colonies of Britain and Germany, Koch increasingly moved from trying to find and identify individual pathogens under the microscope to investigating microbial transmission and susceptibility in larger human and animal populations. The colonial situation, which was characterised by lack of external oversight and individual rights, facilitated this frequently coercive research. In 1900, Koch suspected that malaria outbreaks in New Guinea resulted from changes in the balance between susceptible individuals and carriers. When new non-exposed populations arrived, healthy carriers among the previously exposed population spread the disease to the new arrivals and triggered outbreaks. Koch soon began to think of endemic typhoid in a similar vein, and fully articulated his concept of asymptomatic carriage upon returning to Germany in 1902.[148] [149]

The concept of asymptomatic carriage enabled new ways of tracing and tackling typhoid, but also created ethical dilemma when it came to dealing with the humans unwittingly carrying *S.* Typhi. Public health responses were shaped not just by legal and resource factors, but also by underlying cultural, gender and racial biases about a person's cleanliness and trustworthiness.

Between 1902 and 1906, the Prussian military and Kochian school of bacteriologists embarked on an ultimately futile attempt to eradicate typhoid in areas considered important for Field Marshal Alfred von Schlieffen's plans for an attack on France. This included the mass use of Widal tests and bacteriological culturing to identify and then forcibly isolate and attempt to treat typhoid carriers – an approach that proved unacceptable in German territories outside of the heavily militarised areas of Elsaß and Lothringen.[142] [149] [150] **

** During the interwar period, Norway adopted a similarly radical approach to control typhoid.[151]

British authorities reviewed the German approach. Although they shied away from adopting the draconic style of Prussian microbe hunting, officials employed the new carrier concept to unravel hitherto mysterious typhoid outbreaks.[2] Between 1893 and 1909, the coastal town of Folkestone had suffered from low-level typhoid flare-ups. Officials were aware that most outbreaks were linked to milk, but they failed to find evidence of active infections that might have caused them. Although contaminated milk was traced back to multiple farms, one milker, a Mr N., was found to have worked on all of them during the time of an outbreak. However, N. seemed to be healthy, and it was therefore believed that it was impossible for him to be the source of contagion. In light of the emerging carrier concept, a new medical investigator decided to re-examine the now 60-year-old N. in 1909. Bacteriological examination revealed that N. was an asymptomatic carrier, and had contaminated milk with *S.* Typhi from his faeces. Out of 323 notified local cases between 1896 and 1909, 207 had occurred in houses supplied with milk from a farm where N. worked. While it is unclear what happened to N., it is likely that he had to change his profession and start washing hands not only with water – as he said he did – but also with soap.[152]

The fate of other carriers was markedly worse. There is a long tradition of blaming disease on immigrants, ethnic or religious minorities and poorer working classes. Women were repeatedly singled out by predominantly male medical elites and accused of spreading diseases via ignorance or malevolence.[2] [153] [154] In the history of typhoid, the particularly harsh fate of one working-class, immigrant, minority carrier – who was also a woman – stands out. Her name was Mary Mallon. As with many Irish citizens of her time, Mary had decided to emigrate to the US in 1883. She soon found employment in the New York area and worked as a cook for wealthy families. Although it is unclear when exactly Mary had contracted the initial disease, she was also shedding *S.* Typhi in her stool and infecting her employers. Over the years, a pattern developed: a typhoid outbreak would occur in a family Mary cooked for, but because Mary remained healthy, she would not come under suspicion, and she would use references to find employment with another family, who would eventually also fall prone to the disease. Beginning in 1900, she infected as many as 50 people – several of whom died.[155]

It was only in 1907 that civil engineer George A. Soper identified Mary as the source of an outbreak. Soper had been hired by a family that Mary had cooked for to investigate the source of a typhoid outbreak within their household. After excluding other options, such as defective drains, he began to suspect Mary, who had quit her post three weeks after the outbreak. Soper eventually tracked Mary down after an outbreak in her new employment in a penthouse on Park Avenue in New York City. The encounter at Mary's lodgings must have been dramatic and traumatic. Soper confronted Mary and demanded urine and stool samples to test for typhoid. A frightened and outraged Mary kicked him out. Soper soon returned with the health department and police, who chased Mary down when she attempted to flee. Mary was restrained – with one female inspector sitting on her – and taken to Willard Parker Hospital in New York, where she was forced to provide samples.[155]

Bacteriological examination confirmed that Mary's stool contained *S.* Typhi. In a sign of how uneven bacteriological knowledge had spread, Mary refused to believe that she could be the source of an outbreak. Authorities cited this lack of cooperation as a reason to continue Mary's compulsory quarantine and moved her to Riverside Hospital on North Brother Island just northeast of Manhattan. She was not allowed to leave, had to follow strict hygiene guidelines and was eventually assigned a self-contained small hut to live in. Following failed pharmaceutical interventions, Mary refused offers to surgically attempt to cure her of her infection by removing her gall bladder and tried to regain her freedom by suing the city authorities and paying private laboratories to retest her stool – the samples came back negative. City authorities countered that 120 of the 163 stool samples they had taken had tested positive for typhoid, and that Mary's blood had given a positive reaction with the Widal test. Mary's appeal was rejected in July 1909.[155]

The episode did not go unnoticed by the press. As a result of court proceedings and publications by Soper, Mary became a minor celebrity. US newspapers sensationalised her case and called her 'Typhoid Mary'. Although there were already many other known typhoid carriers, reporters singled out Mary as an 'obstinate' immigrant single woman, who was ignorant of germ theory and had opposed public authorities. Some even tried to visit her on North Brother Island. In a 1909 letter to her lawyer, Mary complained about being made a 'peepshow for everybody'.[155] Her long-term confinement and the curtailment of her rights also raised uncomfortable questions for health authorities. In 1910, a new health commissioner decided to free Mary on the condition that she no longer cook and report back to authorities every few months.

Although her release must have been welcome news for Mary, her new employment as a laundress was far less well paid, and less prestigious. With official supervision lapsing, Mary returned to the better-paid job of cooking in 1914. Using the pseudonyms Mary Brown or Breshoff, she started working for various establishments including the Sloane Maternity Hospital. After causing a typhoid outbreak, which infected 25 people and killed two, she tried to flee but was caught by authorities. This time, quarantine was permanent, and Mary spent the years between 1915 and her death in 1938 (aged 68) living on North Brother Island.[155]

The complex story of 'Typhoid Mary' is indicative of an important transition that typhoid prevention was undergoing around 1900. As a result of broadly effective sanitary interventions and declining case numbers, public health experts were launching increasingly sophisticated campaigns against non-water-related sources of endemic typhoid. Although regulating risky forms of food production proved to be complicated (Chapter 8), officials used a mix of epidemiological and bacterio-logical techniques to hone in on asymptomatic carriers as human reservoirs of *S.* Typhi. Detected carriers were usually trained in hygiene, provided with special sanitary arrangements or told to switch to non-food-related professions. To this day, many countries register and monitor typhoid carriers, who have to agree not to work in sensitive professions involving food preparation or water management.

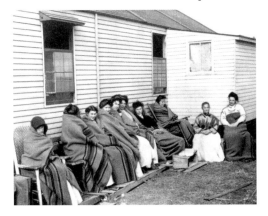

Mary Mallon, better known as Typhoid Mary, sits fourth from the right, among a group of inmates quarantined on North Brother Island in the Long Island Sound.

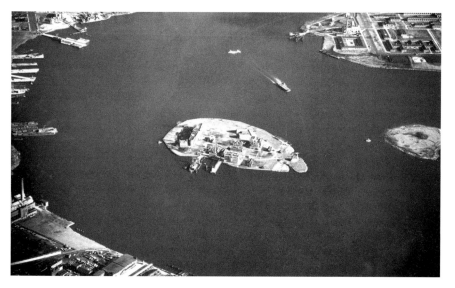

An aerial image of North Brother Island in the Long Island Sound

However, as the case of Mary Mallon shows, not all typhoid carriers were treated equally. In colonial settings, imperial powers' relative neglect of sanitary and public health investment contrasted with the tight-knit surveillance and segregation of 'native populations' in regular contact with white settler populations.[156] [157] In North America and Europe, much depended on a carrier's social and legal status. Although outbreaks were often blamed not on individuals but on faulty sanitary and hygiene arrangements,[2] prevalent stereotypes meant that carriers, who were female or belonged to ethnic or religious minorities, were often treated harsher because they were considered 'dirty', 'obstinate' or 'unable' to adhere to rules. Mallon herself was a complicated character, whose decision to return to work as a cook cost lives. However, New York authorities' treatment of her also revealed many of the prejudices that Irish, Hispanic and Eastern European immigrants faced. Other carriers, who were identified in parallel to Mallon, were allowed to continue their food-related professions after hygiene training.[2] [155] Biased treatment of immigrants was not limited to the US. In interwar Germany, 'Eastern Jews' were considered a dangerous source of diseases such as typhoid and typhus, due to their 'dirty habits'.[158] In Britain, an Italian ice cream vendor was named and shamed for unwittingly spreading typhoid among children in Eccles, while a high-ranking politician was granted anonymity despite causing an outbreak that resulted in 51 deaths.[2] In 2008, the BBC reported that the Long Grove Asylum in Surrey had held female typhoid carriers who were deemed incapable of following hygiene guidance until 1992. Only a few of these women had been sectioned – committed involuntarily to a psychiatric hospital – before being diagnosed with typhoid, and some seem to have been simply forgotten by the system.[159] To this day, minimising infection risks while preventing stigmatisation, discrimination and infringements of carriers' human rights remains a complex challenge in the management of typhoid and many other diseases.

BELOW

Mary Mallon's single-roomed shingled cottage on North Brother Island, with the interior of the cottage shown below it.

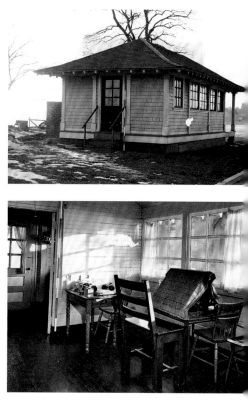

CHAPTER TEN

Vaccination
and vacillation

The effects of the inoculation were jolly unpleasant; we were
in bed for two days with a beastly pain in the side and a sort
of fever. We had to lie on one side all the time ... While it
lasted I think it was the worst thing I have sampled, and if
the genuine article is much worse I hope I shall never get it.

VERE KNIGHT, 1900 [160]

O N THE EVENING of 2 February 1900, Oxford's City Court on St
Aldgate's Street witnessed an unusual gathering. Instead of the usual
crowd of lawyers, prosecutors, witnesses and accused, regimental
physician Dr Hopkinson addressed a group of young men. The men
were part of the British Army's second Oxfordshire Company and were about to
embark for service in Britain's most recent colonial war in South Africa. Following
years of building tensions over the status of non-Dutch-speaking foreigners and
access to the legendary South African gold and diamond fields, war had been declared
in October 1899 against the two independent Boer states of Transvaal and the Orange
Free State. For the British, the first months of the war did not go well. A lightning
offensive of well-armed Boer forces had surprised them, and forced them into a
humiliating retreat, which was followed by Boer sieges of British forts.[161] Amidst
jingoist furore, further troops – among them the Oxfordshire Company – were
dispatched from Britain.

In South Africa, the Oxford men would face both the much-feared partisan
tactics of Boer commandos and a far more lethal enemy in the form of typhoid and
other enteric fevers. Typhoid had only recently been a major cause of death among
US troops sent to attack Spanish possessions during the 1898 Spanish-American
War, and was already causing significant fatalities among British forces in South
Africa.[147] Because it was difficult to provide safe water supplies and adequate
sanitation on the Veldt, British medics were keen to convince reinforcements to
trial a new form of typhoid prevention – vaccination. Speaking to the men gathered
in the Oxford courthouse, Dr Hopkinson stressed that vaccination with the
'typhoid-preventing lymph' would be offered on a voluntary basis. He 'averred that
of those inoculated, only 2.5% succumbed on contracting the disease, while among
those who preferred to remain uninoculated, 9% of the cases proved fatal'.[162]

While it is unclear where exactly Hopkinson had obtained these statistics, it is
clear that his speech failed to convince everybody. During a time of fierce clashes
over compulsory smallpox vaccination, many departing troops refused to be
vaccinated. Some, such as Dr Hopkinson, conflated the killed bacteria on which
typhoid vaccination was based with the 'lymphs' used for smallpox vaccination.

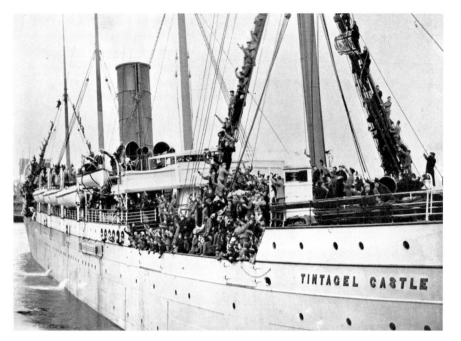

Some, such as W.H. Crumley from the Oxfordshire Light Infantry, who was onboard the *Tintagel Castle* troop transport, did not 'agree'[163] with the principle of vaccination. Others were put off by the side effects, which involved 'beastly pain in the side and a sort of fever'[164] that could incapacitate otherwise healthy young men for several days and was feared to hamper battlefield performance.[165] Finally, some troops may have put off vaccination because typhoid vaccines as a technology were only three years old. Writing to *Jackson's Oxford Journal*, Courtney Brake warned that mass typhoid vaccination was a high-stakes gamble:

> Should the evidence show that it has been useless, a grave responsibility rests upon those who without more adequate data than their own self-confident assumptions have imposed this risky and objectionable ordeal upon our army.[166]

The practice of vaccination itself dates back to the eighteenth century. In 1796, English country physician Edward Jenner* had deliberately infected the eight-year-old son of his gardener with cowpox (or horsepox). Jenner had become intrigued by local folklore, that people who had contracted cowpox did not catch the dreaded smallpox. The experiment worked, and led to the rapid international spread of smallpox vaccination. While Jenner's success was based on anecdotal observations, French microbiologist Louis Pasteur opened the door for a more systematised era of vaccine development and production. In 1879, Pasteur and his co-workers observed that weakened cultures of *Pasteurella multocida* induced immunity against chicken cholera. According to Pasteur's resulting theory of attenuation, weakened but still live pathogens could teach the body to recognise and rapidly respond to bacterial infection. Pasteur and his disciples quickly gained international fame by developing attenuated vaccines against anthrax in 1881, rabies in 1885 and cholera in 1892.[167]

---

* He was not related to royal physician William Jenner, Chapter 3.

The principle of attenuation did not meet with universal acclaim. Convinced that the biological properties of microbial species were unalterable, microbiologists surrounding Robert Koch in Germany had initially rejected the principle of attenuation. Meanwhile, trials with heat-, alcohol- and phenol-killed microbes indicated that it might also be possible to induce immunity using dead microorganisms, which could not regain virulence. In 1896, German and British researchers used these findings to develop the first so-called inactivated vaccines against typhoid.[17] [168]

The two vaccines were developed in parallel to each other. Working as the director of the science section in Robert Koch's Institute for Hygiene in Berlin, bacteriologist Richard Pfeiffer had begun research on Vibrio cholerae (the bacterial cause of cholera) during the early 1890s.[168] [169] As described in Chapter 6, he found that guinea pigs, which had survived an initial injection of Vibrio cholerae, survived further injections of the bacteria. Serum (the fluid component of blood) from surviving guinea pigs agglutinated (clumped together) and destroyed cultures of live V. cholerae. Injecting unexposed guinea pigs with live V. cholerae and the serum of a previously exposed guinea pig protected the unexposed animal. The effect could be replicated in humans who had received a live attenuated cholera vaccine, which had been developed by Waldemar Haffkine in 1892.** As had happened with tests on the guinea pigs, serum from these immunised humans agglutinated cultures of V. cholerae. Both experiments provided strong evidence that a component of serum conferred protection against future infections once a human or animal had survived their first exposure to a live pathogen. The question was whether one could produce a similarly protective serum by injecting inactivated – dead – bacteria.[17] [168] [170]

In 1896, Pfeiffer and his colleague, the bacteriologist Wilhelm Kolle, combined their serum experiments with earlier observations by Pfeiffer – that individual components of bacteria such as the cholera toxin remained active after the original bacterium had been killed – to trial immunisation using inactivated bacteria. S. Typhi was their organism of choice. After identifying a culture suitable for vaccine production with serological agglutination tests (see Chapter 6) in early September 1896, Pfeiffer and Kolle sterilised it by heating it to 56°C and then injected it into two human volunteers. Blood samples were taken before and after the inoculation, and were used to test the protective efficacy of the vaccine in guinea pigs. The results were clear: serum from blood taken before the typhoid inoculation did not protect guinea pigs from exposure to S. Typhi. By contrast, serum from blood taken after the inoculation did protect animals. The inactivated vaccine seemed to protect against live S. Typhi.[17] [168] [170] [172] †

Surprisingly, however, the first person to publish on this new mode of typhoid vaccination was not Pfeiffer or Kolle, but British researcher Almroth Wright.[173] Based at the Army Medical School at Netley, near Southampton, Wright has been

---

** Haffkine's attenuated cholera vaccine was based on the serial passaging of a virulent cholera strain through guinea pigs. He had also used carbolic acid and heat treatment to produce an experimental inactivated vaccine.[168] [171]

† Kolle went on to develop an inactivated whole-cell vaccine for cholera in the same year.

described as a 'Renaissance man'[174] with broad interests. In the field of vaccine development, he had previously conducted research with Waldemar Haffkine on whether a killed V. *cholerae* vaccine could protect guinea pigs against cholera. He had also carried out research on heat-killed vaccines against Malta fever (*Brucella melitensis* – now known as brucellosis), which is a bacterial infection that spreads from animals to humans via unpasteurised dairy products. Initial tests did not go well, and Wright contracted the disease after injecting himself with an experimental vaccine and then testing it by ingesting a culture of live *Brucella*.[168]

At the behest of the Army Medical Department, Wright had commenced research on typhoid vaccination in late 1895. His interest in a heat-killed rather than an attenuated vaccine was piqued following an exchange with Richard Pfeiffer about the latter's observation that exposure to killed *S.* Typhi produced serum that agglutinated live *S.* Typhi. However, in contrast to Pfeiffer and Kolle's focus on protective immunisation, Wright initially seems to have seen the value of inactivated *S.* Typhi injections as a safe way to conduct parallel research on the value of calcium chloride to treat haemorrhages and oedema.[168] [170]

In August 1896, Wright injected a horse with live *S.* Typhi. This resulted in oedema, which disappeared after the horse was given calcium chloride. Another injection of the same horse saw the reappearance but quicker disappearance of the oedema. Together with Army Officer David Semple, Wright trialled a similar procedure on humans. On 31 July 1896, he injected 'M.D.', an officer of the Indian Medical Service, with increasing doses of dead *S.* Typhi while testing the effects of calcium chloride on resulting oedema. Another officer, 'J.S.', was injected with killed *S.* Typhi on 19 August, and his blood was checked for coagulation before and after oral administration of calcium chloride. Serological tests of blood samples taken before and after an injection to assess whether the injection had a protective effect were not conducted. Rather than using heat-killed *S.* Typhi to test immunisation against typhoid – which Kolle and Pfeiffer were doing in Berlin – Wright had designed his experiments to study calcium chloride treatments for oedema. This was also reflected in the title of his *Lancet* paper from 19 September 1896, which was titled 'Association of serous [sic] haemorrhages with conditions of defective blood-coagulability'.[168] [170] [173]

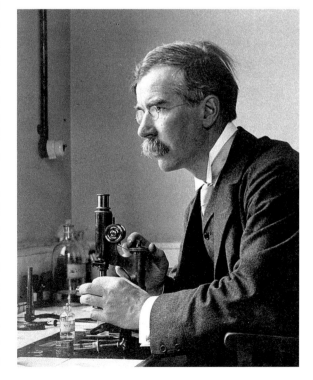

Almroth Wright, c.1900.

Wright's initial focus on oedema treatments began to switch to inducing immunity against typhoid sometime around September 1896. On 25 September – six days after the publication of his *Lancet* paper on calcium chloride – he conducted the first datable experiment explicitly designed to assess the protective efficacy of heat-killed *S.* Typhi by challenging his first volunteer 'M.D.' with a dose of live typhoid bacteria. An additional volunteer received a first dose of heat-killed vaccine on 6 November.[175] But only six days later, on 12 November, Wright must have been dismayed to find that he had been scooped by the publication of Pfeiffer and Kolle's paper on the protective immunisation (Schutzimpfung) of humans against typhoid using heat-killed S. Typhi.[172] Although the publication of the German paper cannot have come as a great surprise given Wright's preceding communication with Pfeiffer, the fact that Pfeiffer and Kolle's trials on humans had only commenced in early September 1896 – and therefore after Wright's first injection of M.D. – would have been irksome.

Wright next tried to salvage his research programme and retake the initiative by increasing the scale and sophistication of his vaccine trials. Within eight days of the publication of the German paper, Wright inoculated 11 new human volunteers – including himself – and began to employ Pfeiffer and Kolle's serological protocol of taking blood before and after an inocculation to assess vaccine efficacy. Rather than start with a discussion of results, his next publication, from 30 January 1897, devoted its first three paragraphs to retrospectively claiming priority for the development of typhoid immunisation with reference to his September 1896 paper, and indirectly accused Pfeiffer of plagiarism.[175] This assertion triggered an ugly priority dispute between German bacteriologists and Wright and his pupils.[17] [168] [170]

Looking back, it is clear that Wright was indeed gravitating towards developing an inactivated typhoid vaccine to immunise humans by late summer 1896. However, he was neither the first to inject heat-killed S. Typhi into humans, nor the first to conduct and publish systematised research on the protective efficacy of inactivated vaccines.[168] [170] While priority for proof of vaccine concept thus rests with the German team, it was Wright's inactivated vaccine that would be the first to be used on a mass basis – and become the most notorious of the first-generation typhoid vaccines.

Wright's military connections were key to the rapid upscaling of his vaccine. With troops based around the world, British military authorities were interested in harnessing the potential benefits of typhoid vaccination. On 30 January 1897, Wright had reported the results of dosing experiments and the successful use of typhoid vaccination to protect himself and further volunteers at Netley from the effects of ingesting live typhoid bacteria. He also proposed using inactivated typhoid vaccines for soldiers going abroad, for health care workers and during epidemics.[175] Wright next tested his vaccine during a real-word typhoid outbreak at the Kent County Asylum, Maidstone, in September 1897. Of 200 members of staff, 84 volunteers were inoculated with the vaccine. None of these volunteers contracted typhoid, while four uninoculated members of staff did. What was not reported in later accounts of the event was that the typhoid outbreak encompassed the entire town – an event that triggered Britain's first use of mass-chlorination (Chapter 7). This meant that uninoculated personnel could have contracted typhoid elsewhere. The inconclusive Maidstone trial was indicative of problems that would engulf Wright's vaccine once larger roll-outs began.[174] [176]

In 1898, Wright organised an additional vaccination trial among British troops while touring India as part of an official plague commission. The inoculation of over 2,800 volunteers occurred without the consent of British authorities, who stopped the trial when they became aware of it. In view of the trial's impromptu nature, there were also problems with guaranteeing that all volunteers received the same vaccine dosage and collecting reliable data on typhoid incidence among vaccinated and unvaccinated control cohorts. Despite this, Wright reported that his vaccine had proven effective. Whereas 2.5 per cent of unvaccinated soldiers had allegedly contracted typhoid, only 0.95 per cent of the vaccinated group had contracted the disease.[17]

In view of these results, Wright received War Office permission to inoculate volunteers heading to South Africa in 1899. Still looking for definitive proof of his vaccine's efficacy, however, Wright once again failed to ensure proper record-keeping of immunisations and of typhoid infections among inoculated and non-inoculated personnel. This not only made it impossible to calculate vaccine efficacy, it also increased distrust when some fully vaccinated soldiers still died of the disease.[174] [176] Although British authorities delivered c.400,000 doses of Wright's vaccine, only c.100,000 soldiers consented to being immunised.[177] ‡ Problems were exacerbated by production and supply-chain issues: some doses had been produced at too high a temperature or stored at the wrong temperature, which diminished their protective efficacy. Because of poor guidance,[178] some clinicians administered too weak or too strong a dose. While underdosing diminished the vaccine's protective effect, overdosing resulted in severer side effects, and may have reduced uptake of the second dose of the vaccine. The fact that Wright's vaccine did not protect against two other enteric fevers (paratyphoid A and B), which were only formally distinguished from typhoid in 1902 but were also circulating among British troops, further contributed to doubts about its effectiveness.[176]

The result of these uncertainties and botched record-keeping was a public relations disaster for Wright's typhoid vaccine. Overall, the Boer War saw about 54,684 reported cases of enteric fever among a mean British Army strength of 208,266. Of the c.22,000 overall British deaths, 8,022 were attributed to enteric fever – a case fatality rate of nearly 15 per cent.[176] Many more non-white troops and civilians, who were caught between the fronts or imprisoned in Britain's anti-insurgency concentration camps, also died of typhoid. Wright subsequently claimed that between five and ten infections had occurred in unvaccinated soldiers for every infection among those who had received his vaccine.[17] However, his repeated failure to ensure adequate statistical follow-up combined with pre-existing anti-vaccination sentiments to produce attacks on his vaccine in the press and the medical establishment. While some celebrities, such as Sherlock Holmes author Arthur Conan Doyle, who had served in a private field hospital during the war, defended typhoid vaccination,[179] others, such as the young Winston Churchill and biologist Alfred Russell Wallace, launched scathing attacks. In his 1904 attempt to evaluate the efficacy of Wright's vaccine, the influential biostatistician – and

An illustration by Archibald Standish Hartrick of a Boer War army medical officer, Joseph Hinton, pulling down the fly of a marquee, in which lie soldiers with enteric fever.

‡ It is unclear whether this number refers to full immunisation with two doses or also includes those who only received one dose.

eugenicist – Karl Pearson highlighted the poor data-gathering and statistical methods employed by Wright, and advised discontinuing vaccination until better proof was forthcoming. The Army's Medical Advisory Board subsequently recommended suspending typhoid vaccination, which had continued on a voluntary basis. In public, Wright, who also prompted controversy with his stringent opposition to women's rights, was mocked as 'Sir Almost Right' or 'Sir Almroth Wrong' – and featured as Sir Colenso Rigeon in George Bernard Shaw's The Doctor's Dilemma.[174] [176]

The Boer War typhoid debacle triggered important reforms within the British armed forces and in the militaries of other countries, who had closely followed events.[145] [177] In Britain, the army established systematised training in sanitation and a programme of screening convalescents to detect new carriers at dedicated enteric depots. Between 1904 and 1909, follow-up investigations by a team surrounding army pathologist and Wright pupil William Leishman led to improvements of typhoid vaccine production and dosage, and also provided statistical proof of the vaccine's protective efficacy.§ Voluntary vaccination was cautiously resumed from 1906 in India – but not for troops on home service.[149] [176]

§ The most important recommendations included the use of the less virulent 'Rawlings strain' (isolated during the Boer War) for all vaccines, and to lower the temperature of sterilisation to 53°C.

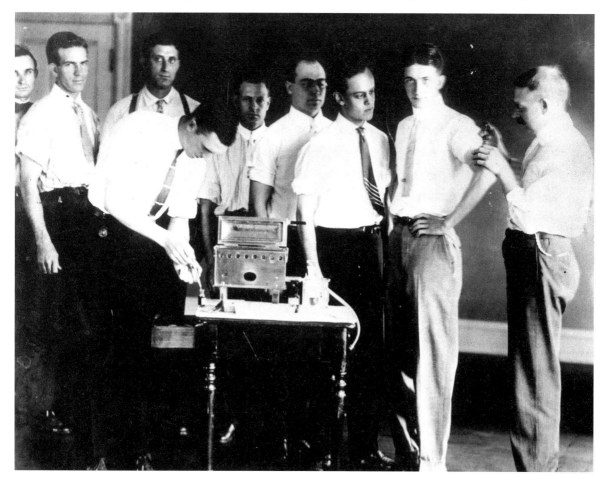

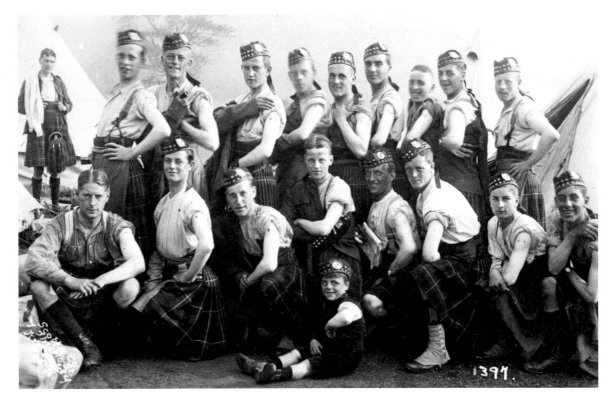

E Company, Liverpool
Scottish Regiment, after
typhoid vaccination, c.1914.

Most other major powers also invested in typhoid vaccines. Between 1904 and 1906, soldiers and settlers in Germany's West African territories were immunised with Pfeiffer and Kolle's typhoid vaccine during the Herero uprising (when Herero and Nama tribes revolted against German colonisers) and subsequent genocide by German troops. In contrast to the British typhoid vaccine, which was administered to the forearm, the German vaccine was administered between nipple and collarbone to minimise irritations. At the behest of typhoid expert Georg Gaffky, vaccination remained voluntary. In an approach similar to that taken by the British, the first dose was administered to troops waiting to embark in Germany, and the second dose was administered on troop ships.[177] In France, voluntary typhoid vaccination was permitted beginning in 1911.[149] [180] In the US, high typhoid rates among troops stationed at home and in the recently occupied Philippines prompted great interest in typhoid vaccination. Initial trials of an oral vaccine took place in 1904, but these were unsuccessful, with volunteers contracting active typhoid fever due to the incomplete inactivation of the so-called Dorset strain of *S. Typhi*.[181] In 1908, Army physician Frederick Russell relaunched development efforts, adapting German and British protocols to produce an improved inactivated typhoid vaccine. After successful human trials in early 1909, a three-dose course of Russell's vaccine was administered on a voluntary basis to over 12,644 members of the US Army by 1911. Accurate record-keeping showed that only five cases of typhoid occurred after full vaccination. The positive data prompted the US armed forces to introduce compulsory typhoid vaccination in the same year.[181]–[184]

During the First World War, all of the major powers tried to protect their troops from typhoid with a mix of sanitation and vaccination. The decision about whether

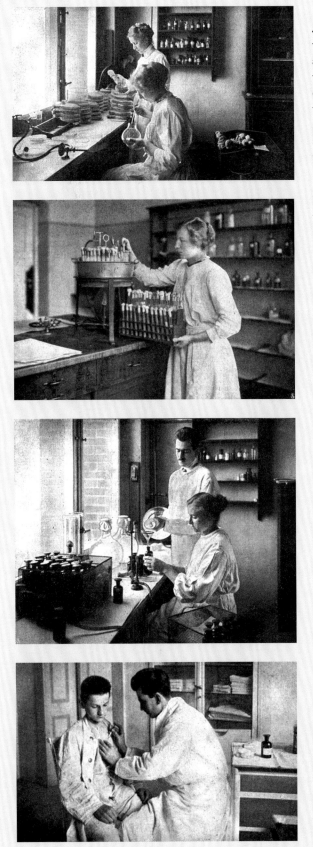

A GROWING NUMBER of major powers began to use killed 'whole-cell vaccines'. However, production methods and the bacterial strains used for the vaccine varied. In Britain, Wright had initially employed a broth technique, whereby virulent typhoid bacteria were grown for 2–3 weeks at 39°C and then killed at 60°C, after which, sterilising Lysol was added up to a concentration of 0.5%. Investigations by Leischman subsequently led to inactivation at 53°C. The Germans initially employed a Kochian agar-based approach to grow the bacteria, which were then rinsed off with saline solution and killed at between 60 and 65°C, after which, 3% carbolic acid was added against contamination.[177] In the US, Russell used the agglutinating power of rabbit serum as an index of immunity, which made him decide to combine the agar- and broth-based culturing methods, and to lower the temperature used to kill bacteria to 53°C, which were then stored in saline solution with 0.25% tricresol added to prevent contamination. He also advocated vaccine production in smaller batches to achieve more uniform inactivation and use of the less virulent 'Rawlings strain' which had been isolated from a British soldier during the Boer War.[17] [182] Other researchers produced experimental vaccines using different temperatures, or by using chemicals such as phenol to kill cultures. Dosages, and the recommended number of vaccine doses, also varied. Whereas British and German troops received two doses, the US Army increased the number of doses to three. French soldiers initially received four doses, before wartime constraints led to a reduction of the number of doses to two (with a higher concentration per dose).[180]

LEFT, FROM TOP
German vaccine production, c.1915: (1) typhoid bacteria are grown on culture medium, (2) the bacteria are killed by placing vials in a heated water bath, (3) solutions of killed bacteria are diluted, (4) the vaccine is administered.

to roll out vaccines on a compulsory or voluntary basis reflected different societies' value systems and historical experiences with vaccination. In France, memories of the Franco-Prussian War (where France had suffered far larger losses from smallpox than had the vaccinated Prussian troops) led to compulsory typhoid vaccination of army (but not navy) recruits upon enrolment – although coverage remained well below 80 per cent.[149] [180] Early German coverage rates were even patchier. Although planners saw the war as a chance to test different vaccine types, many army members tried to avoid the unpleasant experience of vaccination. It was only following the establishment of trench warfare and high disease losses among non-immunised troops during the first eight months of the war that commanders launched a more vigorous vaccination campaign, in 1915.[176] [180] [185]–[187] A similar story occurred in Austria-Hungary, where military command had initially banned typhoid vaccines for fear of adverse reactions that might have slowed mobilisation, but they soon reversed this decision in the face of mass outbreaks.[182] [188] In Russia, the tsarist government also introduced mandatory vaccinations in August 1915, but troops still suffered from comparatively high levels of disease. After 1918, Soviet officials, who were keen to highlight tsarist failures alongside the advantages of preventive socialist health, launched mass campaigns of smallpox and typhoid vaccination.[180] [189]

In contrast to their French and American allies, British authorities relied on a programme of voluntary vaccination. Britain's decision not to implement compulsory vaccination was based on a mix of factors. These related to Britain's liberal political traditions, recent popular protest against compulsory vaccination, as well as memories of the Boer War roll-out. With hundreds of thousands of volunteers enrolling in the army in 1914, prominent spokespeople attempted to ensure high vaccine uptake. Public supporters included Almroth Wright, William Osler (a founding member of Johns Hopkins University, and subsequently Regius Professor of Medicine at Oxford) and Lord Kitchener (Secretary of State for War and Commander-in-Chief during the latter stages of the Boer War). Vaccine proponents argued that sanitation on the battlefield would be limited, and that it was soldiers' patriotic duty to get vaccinated to protect themselves and defeat the Germans. Trying to tap into the nationalist furore of 1914, Kitchener even declared that vaccine refusers would not be sent abroad.

Anti-vaccination activists did not back down easily. Although the number of active campaigners seems to have been relatively small, they made effective use of mass-distributed pamphlets as well as columns, articles and letters in popular magazines and newspapers. Emboldened by their recent success in gaining the right to conscientiously object to smallpox vaccination in 1907, British anti-vaccination activists challenged the principles of germ theory, which some described as a dangerous German science, warned of threats to British liberal values and highlighted alleged adverse effects and fatalities resulting from vaccination.[149] [176]

The result was a public battle for vaccine uptake. Although only 25–30 per cent of the British Expeditionary Force arriving in France were fully immunised against typhoid in the autumn of 1914, numbers surged to 90–98 per cent as a result of a hasty one-shot immunisation campaign, but they dropped again soon afterwards. In early 1915, Osler accused 'misguided cranks' of sabotaging the British war effort,

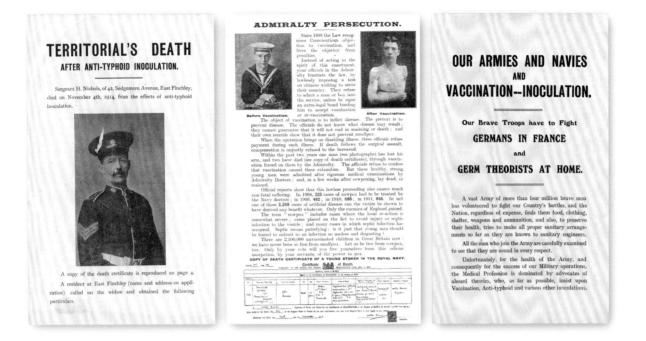

The First World War saw significant campaigning by anti-vaccine activists against the voluntary roll-out of typhoid vaccinations among British troops. Pamphlets alleged deaths and amputations resulting from typhoid vaccination, and tried to portray the vaccine as a dangerous product of German bacteriology c.1914–18.

and the army issued pamphlets supporting vaccination. By late 1916, around 90 per cent of British soldiers were vaccinated. As a result of high vaccination rates and a strong focus on sanitation, typhoid fatalities remained comparatively low among all major powers throughout the war.[149] [176]

Inactivated typhoid vaccines' wartime success did not translate into popularity among civilian populations. While some countries, such as France, tried to integrate typhoid vaccines into emerging immunisation schedules, most post-war governments did not consider mass typhoid vaccination suitable for non-emergency use.[149] The reasons for this were manifold: vaccine side effects put many people off from receiving their first or returning for a second dose; the ongoing decline of wider typhoid rates led to complacency; and in countries such as Germany, authorities noted a general peacetime vaccine exhaustion after intensive wartime campaigns. [142] Meanwhile, populations that were at particular risk, such as close contacts of carriers, doctors and nurses, troops going abroad, merchant seamen, travellers and colonial settlers, could still access vaccines.[180]

With the advantage of hindsight, the advent of vaccination in 1896 can thus be seen as an extension of, rather than a revolution of, existing sanitary practices.[149] Beginning in the 1870s, investigations into typhoid's environmental spread had led to the design of increasingly effective interventions to stop waterborne transmission, improve food safety and minimise the public health risks posed by chronic carriers. Vaccines were used as an additional safeguard against typhoid for at-risk populations, during emergencies and outbreaks and in areas where sanitation was unavailable. In contrast to popular tales of heroic sanitary awakenings or bacteriological revolutions, none of these interventions had evolved in a straight-forward manner, and none would have been able to effectively combat typhoid by themselves. However, in combination with increasingly fine-grained disease surveillance, they formed a toolkit that not only opened the way for typhoid control but – by the 1940s (Chapter 12) – increasingly held out the prospect for eventual elimination.

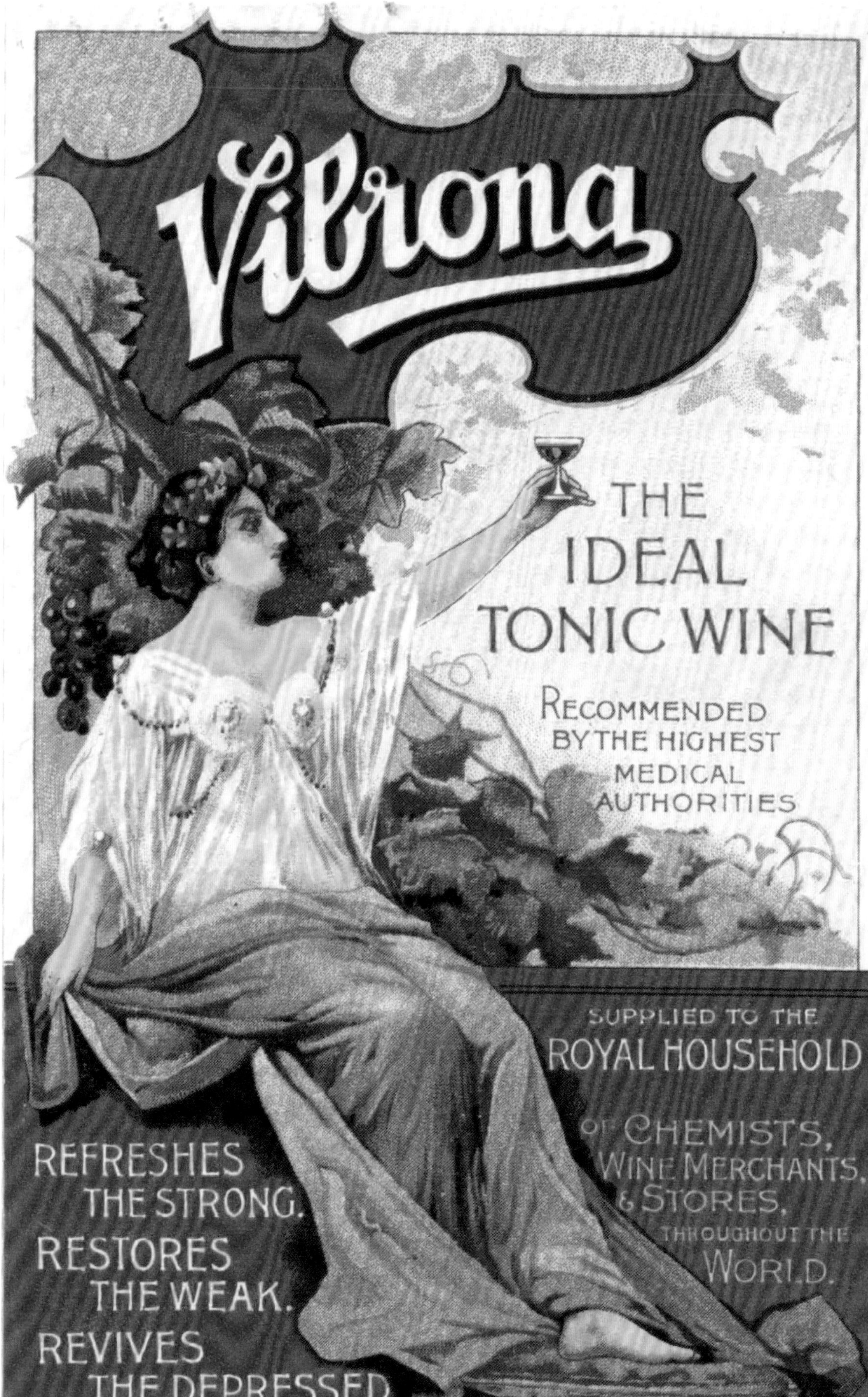
Vibrona
THE
IDEAL
TONIC WINE
RECOMMENDED
BY THE HIGHEST
MEDICAL
AUTHORITIES
SUPPLIED TO THE
ROYAL HOUSEHOLD
OF CHEMISTS,
WINE MERCHANTS,
& STORES,
THROUGHOUT THE
WORLD.
REFRESHES
THE STRONG.
RESTORES
THE WEAK.
REVIVES
THE DEPRESSED.

CHAPTER ELEVEN

Asepsis, antipyresis and antibiotics

During the prevalence of Typhoid Fever, Bubonic Plague, Cholera, and Small Pox. Do not fail to have packets of 'Petal Dust,' freely distributed in the house ... 'Petal Dust' will ozonise much of the atmospheric oxygen, and render the danger of infection from all contagious diseases infinitesimal.

ROSMARINE MANUFACTURING CO., LONDON, C.1891

Through a severe attack of Typhoid Fever last March I rapidly lost my hair ... Then I saw your advertisement and it seemed so reasonable that I commenced taking Capsuloids. First they acted as a marvellous tonic. Very soon the falling out ceased, and they toned me up as well as my hair ...

THE CAPSULOID COMPANY, LTD, LONDON, 1904

Kerol is the best general disinfectant. Use it for drains, sinks ... Use it in the sick-room – for it prevents infection from such contagious diseases as diphtheria, typhoid, cholera, scarlatina, and measles, Use it in the bath ... Use it as a gargle ... Use it for the hair ... Use it as an animal wash; Use it as a garden spray; Use it everywhere and anywhere...

QUIBELL BROS. LTD, C.1910

A CENTURY after Pierre-Charles-Alexandre Louis first established the modern disease category of typhoid fever (Chapter 3), powerful tools had been developed to track *S.* Typhi, and to stop it from spreading between human bodies. However, virtually no tools existed to combat the bacterium once it had entered a body. All one could do was hope that the disease would run its course without killing or maiming the patient. The absence of a proven cure did not mean that doctors, patients and families remained passive. Around the world, physicians experimented with treatments to combat typhoid and fortify immune systems. Meanwhile, families and patients could purchase a wide array of commercial treatments – none of which worked, and some of which could cause harm.

Interventions reflected the crowded marketplace of humoral, contagionist and anti-contagionist explanations of disease, and were often based on a hybrid of existing theories. During the 1820s, Louis had disparaged contemporary physicians'

OPPOSITE
An advertisement for Vibrona Tonic Wine, billed as a restorative for victims of typhoid fever, 1891.

excessive use of bloodletting and purgatives to treat fevers. However, in his own treatment of typhoid fever, he also relied on a mix of symptomatic interventions, ranging from blood-letting to restorative diets, infusions of cinchona bark, barley water, whey and flaxseed, tonics, aromatic wine and camphorated alcohol.[22]

Louis was not alone in placing a special emphasis on patients' diets. Because typhoid was classified as a fever and diarrhoeal disease, many nineteenth-century physicians tried to counteract its effects by starving the fever and administering restorative fluids. Prescribed liquid diets ranged from fortified milk and bouillon to copious amounts of alcohol. While these diets likely exacerbated many a patient's condition, the late nineteenth century saw a gradual shift of dietary advice towards nutritious solid foods, including porridges, stews, meats and bananas.[190]–[192] Despite growing controversies about the extent of its use,[193] milk continued to play a prominent dietary role, with at least 1.5 litres (3 pints) per day administered to patients who were unable to eat anything. Guaranteeing a safe and regular supply caused much debate among physicians working in tropical environments. They also reported having to supplement restorative diets with 'the accustomed whisky, cocktail or any champagne mixture'[177] to avoid withdrawal symptoms among their heavy-drinking European patients. In accordance with the racial paradigms of the era, white patients were supposed to be nursed by white personnel. 'Indigenous patients' were to be treated according to 'native' customs.[177]

Trying to lower a patient's fever formed a second point of attack. As a result of contemporary physiological research and the spread of medical thermometers (Chapter 6), a growing number of practitioners reported that a reduction in a patient's fever preceded an improvement of other symptoms. This prompted many to artificially reduce fevers with aggressive antipyretic treatments. In German-speaking areas, cold-water baths and hydrotherapy proved particularly popular as a way to lower fevers, restore 'nervous energy' and stop tissue deterioration. Administering quinine, calomel, iodine and digitalis to control fevers proved similarly popular. In 1874, the discovery that salicylic acid (the substance behind aspirin's anti-inflammatory action) also appeared to reduce fevers prompted growing interest in chemical antipyresis. Salicylic acid could be produced cheaply in large quantities and soon proved popular for the treatment of typhoid – despite significant side effects.[194]

The advent of germ theory and increasing acknowledgement of typhoid's contagious properties also led doctors to experiment with antiseptic treatments. During the 1850s, William Budd had already advocated disinfecting patients' rooms, toilets and faeces to destroy the typhoid 'poison' (Chapter 7). With British surgeon Joseph Lister promoting the use of carbolic acid to disinfect surgical instruments, wounds and hands beginning in the 1860s, other practitioners began to use disinfectants as internal treatments. In addition to salicylic and carbolic acid, some doctors prescribed the ingestion of magnesium sulphate, salol and copious amounts of hot water.[194]–[196] None of these interventions was safe, effective or pleasant.

Doctors were not the only ones devising new treatments. The rise of lucrative markets for mass-produced substances such as salicylic acid opened the door for an increasing professionalisation of pharmaceutical research, development and marketing. Although understandings of metabolic pathways and disease aetiology continued to vary, the late nineteenth century saw large chemical manufacturers draw on advances in biochemistry to try and replace 'natural' substances such as quinine and opium with synthetic alkaloids for use against fever or pain. Emerging pharmaceutical giants, such as aspirin manufacturer Bayer, soon began to sell trademarked therapeutic substances across multiple continents.[194] [197] [198]

The new mass-produced pharmaceuticals entered an already crowded marketplace of diets, drugs and medical devices. In the absence of significant state regulation, patients could purchase trademarked pharmaceutical substances alongside various other pills, tonics or injections. Some doctors would prescribe and prepare their own drugs – often with a hefty markup. Others would send patients to pharmacists, who would prepare drugs according to a doctor's prescription but would also sell therapeutics based on pharmacopoeias or their own recipes. In colonial settings, government-authorised dispensaries were another important source of active pharmaceutical substances. Across the world, medical consumers could also turn to a wide array of elaborately marketed patent remedies that were sold over the counter or by itinerant traders. The secretive nature of the ingredients and exaggerated claims that often accompanied them helped give rise to the term 'snake oil salesman'. There were also flourishing markets for homeopathic treatments, various vernacular medical traditions and faith-based interventions. With so many treatment options to choose from and no controlled clinical trials to evaluate safety and efficacy, it is unsurprising that many patients decided to mix and match.[198]–[201]

In the case of typhoid, turn-of-the-century magazines, newspapers and bill-boards were full of advertisements for remedies promising miraculous cures or restorative treatments. Although few guaranteed actual cures for typhoid, many promised protection and rapid recovery. Around 1900, British consumers could

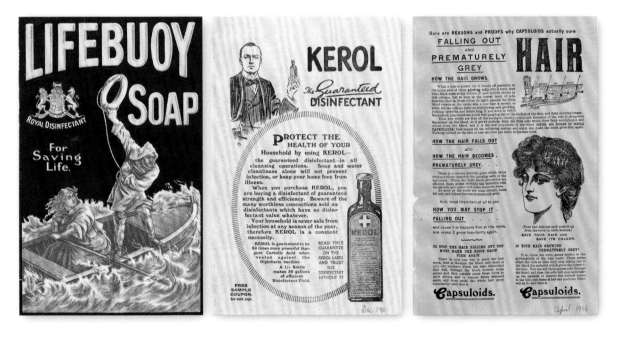

purchase rose-petal dust (to disinfect 'tainted' air), capsuloids (to purify the blood or restore hair), disinfectants and soaps for internal and external use, and dietary supplements to aid recovery. Victorian consumers, who were distrustful of their local water supply, could also buy a range of household and pocket-sized water filters, which contained charcoal as an active ingredient.

Although manufacturers no longer advertise curative properties, some of these products, such as tonic wines, Eno's Fruit Salts and Sanitas, are still with us. Eno's fruit-derived salts were first sold by British pharmacist James Crossley Eno as a 'natural health-giving agent' in 1852. Advertisements claimed that the salts were effective against fevers and poisons, and roused the spirits.[202] [203] While these therapeutic claims have long since been debunked, Eno salts remain popular as an antacid in India. The disinfectant Sanitas was similarly advertised as a non-poisonous typhoid preventative that could be used at different doses to treat water, preserve beer, meat and milk, and disinfect roads, urinals and floors. Some consumers allegedly drank diluted Sanitas to prevent internal infection. Manufacturers claimed that Sanitas worked by dispelling foul odour and – after the spread of germ theory – bacteria. The product had originated in the 1870s as a result of contemporaries' equation of the 'therapeutic' aroma of pine forests with the aseptic odour and properties of hydrogen peroxide – the smell of which still pervades modern bathrooms.[204] [205]

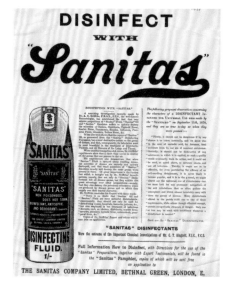

An advertisement for Sanitas, which was billed as an external and internal disinfectant, 1891.

Unfortunately, effective typhoid cures remained elusive even after germ theory had become more widely accepted and vaccines emerged. In the case of healthy carriers, doctors tried in vain to eliminate *S.* Typhi from bodies by repurposing substances, such as urotropine and Brewer's yeast, that were used for other digestive and urinary disorders.[206] Surgeons also attempted to eliminate the source of infection by removing carriers' gall bladders. The success rate of these cholecystectomies was mixed and undoubtedly contributed to fear amongst carriers such as Mary Mallon, who refused the procedure (Chapter 9). Between the 1920s and 1950s, there were also attempts to use bacteria-infecting viruses (bacteriophages), therapeutic vaccines and serum therapies (Chapter 6) to treat and prevent typhoid. All of these, however, failed to perform reliably in clinical trials, and were gradually phased out.[206]–[208]

An advertisement for Eno's Fruit Salts, 1911.

It was only in 1948 that the first effective therapy for typhoid emerged, in the form of the antibiotic chloramphenicol (chloromycetin). Starting in the 1930s, targeted research to find chemical and biological compounds capable of killing or neutralising bacterial cells while leaving human cells unharmed had given rise to a growing number of effective antimicrobial drugs. Chloramphenicol, which is produced by *Streptomyces venezuelae*, was first isolated in 1947 by scientists working for American pharmaceutical company Parke-Davis.[209] To test potential appli-

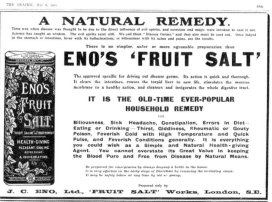

cations of the drug, Parke-Davis provided samples to doctors treating various infectious diseases. Chloramphenicol's effectiveness against the disease scrub typhus, which is caused by the bacterium *Orientia tsutsugamushi* and was a major concern in warzones, had already become apparent during early laboratory and human trials. To provide further evidence, a team of experts from the US Army and the University of Maryland was issued with batches of chloramphenicol and sent to Malaysia in 1948. Members of the team included the clinician Theodore E. Woodward, who had been part of the US Army Typhus Commission, as well as future FDA commissioner Herbert Ley Jr, who was part of the Army Epidemiology Board.[210] [211]

The team reached Kuala Lumpur during the so-called 'Malay Emergency', which saw armed conflict break out between the communist Malayan National Liberation Army and the British colonial government supported by Malayan police troops. The US team began to make promising progress in using chloramphenicol to treat victims of scrub typhus. Woodward treated 40 patients with clinical signs of scrub typhus, which included 30 with confirmed scrub typhus and 10 with other diseases

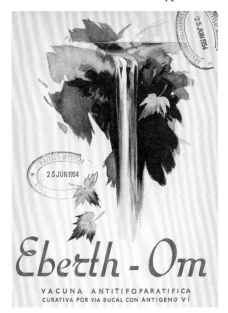

An advertisement for an allegedly therapeutic oral typhoid and paratyphoid vaccine called Eberth-Om, Estudio Om, 1953.

that caused a similar clinical picture. The latter group included one patient from a rubber plantation, who had arrived alongside a later-confirmed scrub typhus case one Saturday night and had to be examined by candlelight prior to treatment. The patient did not have skin lesions (eschars) that indicated bites by mites, but had a toxic appearance. While his colleague's fever subsided within 24 hours of chloramphenicol treatment, the patient's condition persisted, and was accompanied by abdominal distress and diarrhoea. Further tests confirmed the presence of *S.* Typhi. Remarkably, however, his symptoms began to improve within 48 hours of starting chloramphenicol treatment, and his fever disappeared within 72 hours. Treatment was interrupted on the fifth day because of concerns about wasting precious chloramphenicol on an infection that was beyond the remit of the US team's research mission, but was resumed after the patient relapsed on the eighth day. Another confirmed typhoid patient recovered within four days of receiving chloramphenicol. Further trials were subsequently carried out in the US.[210] [211]

Published between 1948 and 1950, news of chloramphenicol's effectiveness against *S.* Typhi was celebrated as evidence of a miraculous new age of antibiotic treatment. Some 119 years after Louis had set out a pathological definition of typhoid fever, a cure for the dreaded disease had finally been found. Bacterial resistance against chloramphenicol would soon surface and the drug did not prevent or resolve the carrier state (Chapter 13).* However, experts were confident that the combination of sanitation, food hygiene, vaccines, carrier control and a steady stream of new antibiotics would not only control but enable the elimination of typhoid – at least on a regional basis.

---

* Licensed in 1961, ampicillin showed greater efficacy in the treatment of carriers. Mixing high doses of other antibiotic treatments with cholecystectomy also proved effective.[212]

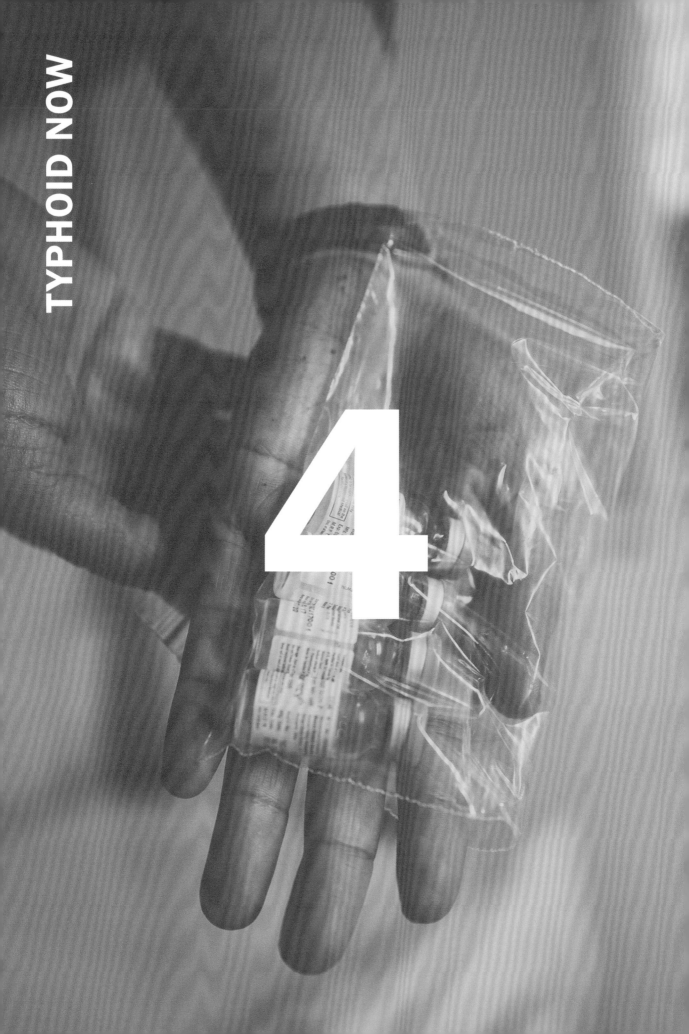

4

> We were vaccinated – and obviously we didn't know whether we were getting the new typhoid vaccine they were testing, the existing typhoid vaccine that's approved in the UK, and the placebo which was a meningitis vaccine, and then … we were invited to down a shot of typhoid.
>
> DAINA, 2019, INTERVIEW FOR TYPHOIDLAND

Between 2015 and 2016, 112 volunteers cycled, walked and drove up Oxford's Headington Hill to take part in a clinical trial. Once they reached the Churchill Hospital, one group received a meningitis vaccine, a second group received an already licensed typhoid vaccine and a third group received a new typhoid conjugate vaccine (TCV). Neither the participants nor the nurses administering the vaccines knew which was which. The next time the volunteers arrived, they drank two vials of fluid. The first contained bicarbonate to neutralise their stomach acid, and the second contained live *S*. Typhi bacteria suspended in further bicarbonate. While participants later disagreed on whether the typhoid vial tasted differently, they all agreed that drinking bicarbonate was vile. Over subsequent weeks, volunteers returned for regular checks and delivered stool and blood samples for bacteriological analysis. At the first sign of an infection, they were placed on a course of antibiotics. When the anonymised trial data were unblinded in late 2017, a clear picture emerged: TCV was well-tolerated, safe and had a significant protective effect. According to the Oxford trial lead, Andrew Pollard, the TCV vaccine would 'be a real game-changer'.[213] But why was another game-changer necessary? Hadn't the development of sanitation, older vaccines, antibiotics and public health surveillance provided a powerful toolkit to control typhoid? In this final part of the book, we will explore how global inequality first led to a neglect of typhoid, and how this neglect facilitated a resurgence of increasingly drug-resistant typhoid.

OPPOSITE
Health worker holding four vials of the new Typhoid Conjugate Vaccine (TCV), 2021.

CHAPTER TWELVE

An ancient disease
of exotic places

The public health authorities are now in a position to ...
intensify the campaign against the chronic carrier. It appears
to be possible to devise a long-term policy ... that might in
time lead to the complete eradication of enteric infection.

ARTHUR FELIX, 1951[214]

For most typhoid experts, the years after 1945 were ones of unprecedented optimism. Although the wartime breakdown of sanitation and public health led to a temporary resurgence of typhoid fever across Europe and Japan, commentators in richer countries believed that the time was close to move from disease control to eradication.

Experts' confidence was based on the effectiveness of sanitation, vaccines and antibiotics in reducing typhoid infections, as well as on recent breakthroughs in microbiologists' ability to identify the 'unextinguished residuum' of typhoid within their populations.

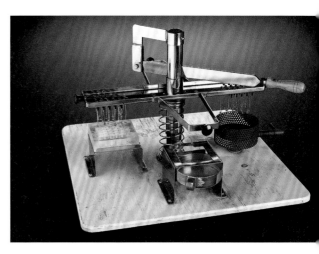

Phage-typing machine, London, 1959. By the early 1950s, phage-typing had become mechanised to speed processing. A machine could simultaneously apply 29 drops of bacteriophage filtrate to a bacterial culture under investigation.

Using a technology called bacteriophage-typing, which employs standardised sets of bacteria-infecting viruses (bacteriophages) to distinguish between different strains of *S.* Typhi, microbiologists were able to link and trace sporadic typhoid outbreaks back to carriers. During the Second World War, microbiologist Arthur Felix at Britain's Emergency Public Health Laboratory Service (EPHLS) had begun to use bacterio-phage-typing to investigate typhoid outbreaks across the country, and to build a 'fingerprint' registry of the different *S.* Typhi types excreted by chronic carriers.* In case of an outbreak, authorities could quickly check whether the isolated phage type of *S.* Typhi matched those shed by local carriers.[214]–[217]

The fingerprinting programme was a sweeping success. Across the country, seemingly random typhoid outbreaks were shown to be linked. Between 1941 and 1942, authorities in Hertfordshire and Buckinghamshire had detected a series of seemingly unrelated typhoid cases. Centralised data pooling not only showed that all of the widely dispersed cases had been caused by the rare phage type D4, it also traced their origin back through milk depots to a farm, which was located 100 miles away, in the county of Wiltshire. The carrier was a farmer, who was unaware of ever having contracted typhoid. He had passed *S.* Typhi onto customers via

---

* Felix was a world authority on typhoid and had co-discovered the O (somatic) and H (flagellar) antigens (1915/16) and the Vi (capsular) antigen (1934), which led to Vi-serodiagnostics for carriers (Chapter 6).

unpasteurised milk, which was sometimes mixed with pasteurised milk in centralised depots. According to EPHLS investigators, pooling epidemiological and phage-typing data could identify carriers 'no less precisely than can be the criminal by his fingerprint'.[218]

Combined with new selective media and gauze (Moore) swabs for sewage outlets, phage-typing could even solve complex outbreaks involving contaminated watercourses. In 1944, two boys, 15 and 17 years old, were taken ill with suspected typhoid fever at Helmington Row Hospital in Crook. Three secondary cases were subsequently reported, and one of the boys died of the disease. Public health authorities found that all S. Typhi strains belonged to the same phage type A, and that both boys had attended a Whit Monday excursion organised by Hunwick Sunday School. Questioning revealed that the group had set off to Barnard Castle by train and then hiked up to Lartington, where they had lunch. It was a hot day, and some members of the group – among them, the two boys – had decided to spend the remainder of the day by the River Balder. Despite warnings, the boys had used river water to make lemonade. Unbeknownst to them, they had taken water from just 60 yards below the main sewage outlet of the 600-inhabitant village of Cotherstone. Subsequent analysis of river and sewage water revealed high concentrations of S. Typhi phage type A. Investigators next examined local medical records, and found that one 76-year-old woman had suffered from typhoid fever while in India in 1936. Bacteriological examination revealed that she was a chronic carrier, whose phage type matched those of the outbreaks. Authorities subsequently provided her with special means for sewage disposal.[219] [220]

With microbiologists across Europe, North America, Australia and Japan adopting phage-typing, researchers became increasingly interested in how to distinguish 'native' from 'foreign' typhoid types. The aim was both to understand microbiological diversity and to quickly react to the introduction of new typhoid types into areas with low incidence. Concerned about typhoid carriers among demobilised service personnel, British authorities had already advocated mandatory screening of returning army and navy personnel in 1944. Following the end of the war, the resumption of civilian travel, mass labour migration and tourism heightened concerns. By the 1950s, microbiologists from both sides of the Iron Curtain collaborated to map the global diversity of S. Typhi.[216]

International collaboration could lead to spectacular public health triumphs. During the winter of 1963, 177 inhabitants and 260 tourists visiting the famous Swiss ski resort of Zermatt developed typhoid, with three resulting deaths. Local clinicians initially confused typhoid symptoms with a parallel outbreak of influenza. However, the outbreak was picked up by surveillance in the UK, which detected a spike of S. Typhi phage type E1 in returning tourists. Subsequent Swiss investigations revealed two probable points of

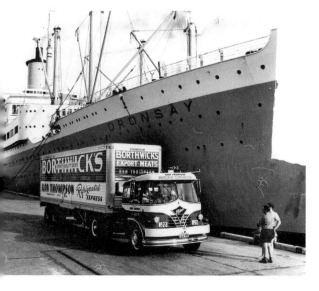

The SS *Oronsay* at Brisbane Wharf, prior to 1955.

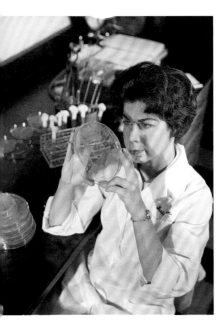

pollution, resulting from the faecal contamination of the town's water source by either a 20-year-old Italian miner or a sewage leak. In both scenarios, defective chlorination had enabled the subsequent outbreak.[221] Seven years later, phage-typing was able to unravel a mass typhoid outbreak among 83 crew members and passengers aboard the cruiser SS Oronsay. The outbreak had been caused by a strain of S. Typhi that was common on the Indian subcontinent. In addition to revealing gross accommodation disparities for European and non-European crew, investigations discovered two asymptomatic carriers among the Goanese crew, and multiple related cases in the many ports at which the SS Oronsay had called during its voyage from Southampton to Vancouver.[222]

Unfortunately, the benefits of public health breakthroughs remained unevenly distributed. While inhabitants of wealthier countries had never enjoyed greater protection from S. Typhi, typhoid remained a major killer outside of their borders. Resource constraints, political instability, lack of access to sanitary and health services and growing pressure on water resources meant that poorer areas around the world continued to suffer from high typhoid burdens.

Wealthy countries did little to change this. Despite developing sophisticated sampling networks to map S. Typhi diversity, the primary aim of these systems was to stop 'the dangers of an invasion of typhoid fever in Europe and North America'.[223] Microbiologists' research priorities reflected and reinforced growing political concerns about migration. Whereas US authorities focused on identifying Mexican and, increasingly, Vietnamese typhoid types, British authorities focused on typhoid types originating in the Indian subcontinent, and French authorities focused on Africa and Oceania.[216]

This shift towards trying to map and stop foreign strains from crossing borders had multiple consequences. Whereas typhoid had once been viewed as a universal threat, wealthy countries' success in containing its spread increasingly changed its popular image, into that of a 'foreign' disease threat waiting to reinvade cleansed territories. Although individual outbreaks continued to occur,[224] fading memories of typhoid as a domestic disease of filth (Chapter 4) were replaced with concepts of typhoid as a disease of 'backward' places. As long as it stayed there, the ongoing circulation of S. Typhi triggered little international action.

Safe water, sanitation, vaccines and antibiotics remained unavailable in many parts of the world. This Chinese Ministry of Health poster from 1951 depicts S. Typhi and a typhoid victim, describes symptoms, advises good nursing and warns about death resulting from intestinal bleeding.

② 傷寒大都在秋天發病，開始時經覺疲憊、頭重、胃口不好和有點發冷，幾天以後，發熱越來越高，連着兩三個星期，日夜不退，有的說糊話，認不得人，這是腸子裏裹潰的毛病，如果調養得不好，腸子出血或爛穿，就會有生命危險。

CHAPTER THIRTEEN
Losing control

It would be a disaster, therefore, if the reckless use of antibiotics in animal or human medicine resulted in the transmission of chloramphenicol resistance to *S.* Typhi with sufficient frequency to become epidemiologically important.

E.S. ANDERSON, 1968[225]

WEALTHY COUNTRIES' reconceptualisation of typhoid as a 'foreign' disease was mirrored at the international level of politics. With major donors such as the USA prioritising other diseases, such as malaria and smallpox, UN agencies did not devote much attention to typhoid.[226] Although the disease was acknowledged as a concern of the 'developing world', flare-ups of attention were brief. During the 1950s, several international reports focused on post-war epidemics in Europe and re-evaluating the efficacy of existing typhoid vaccines. A second and third wave of attention occurred around 1970 and 2000 – this time as a result of disturbing reports about new antibiotic-resistant strains of *S.* Typhi.

ANTIMICROBIAL RESISTANCE
Around 1964, an Israeli typhoid patient at the Assaf Harofe Government Hospital on the outskirts of Tel Aviv had their gallbladder removed. By itself, this was nothing unusual. The young state of Israel had experienced high levels of endemic typhoid during the 1950s, which resulted in some of those infected becoming asymptomatic carriers.[227] What was uncommon was that cholecystectomy and two years of repeated treatment with high doses of different antibiotics failed to eliminate *S.* Typhi from the patient's body. During a second hospitalisation due to typhoid cholangitis, *S.* Typhi strains isolated from the patient proved resistant to multiple antibiotics. Worryingly, isolates' ability to resist different antibiotics was encoded on multiple plasmids – small circular strands of DNA – that can be exchanged between bacteria.[228]

The phenomenon of antimicrobial resistance (AMR) is not specific to typhoid, and pre-dates the development of modern antibiotics by millennia. Antibiotics work by inhibiting the growth of bacteria, or by killing bacteria altogether. Microorganisms themselves produce and use antimicrobial substances to gain evolutionary advantages. Some bacteria are naturally resistant to the effects of certain antibiotics. Others can develop the ability to resist antibiotics with random mutations, or by acquiring AMR genes from the environment (transformation), via bacteriophages (transduction) or by exchanging AMR genes (conjugation) with other bacteria. The latter three mechanisms are also referred to as horizontal gene transfer.[229]

The fact that *S.* Typhi could rapidly develop mutational resistance against individual antibiotics like chloramphenicol or ampicillin – which had entered the global market in 1961 – was already well-known by the mid-1960s. In 1950, two years after chloramphenicol had first been used against typhoid in Malaya, physicians in the British city of Sheffield had reported that *S.* Typhi isolates from a 43-year-old patient had become increasingly resistant to chloramphenicol over the course of treatment.[230] However, in an age of rapid antibiotic innovation, most observers remained confident that increased dosages and new drugs would be able to stay ahead of AMR. This prediction was over-optimistic.

Between 1959 and 1965, Japanese and British research on the transfer of multiple drug resistance (MDR) amongst and between different bacteria species highlighted that AMR was an 'infective' genetic trait that could spread rapidly through microbial populations.[231] The new scenarios of 'infective resistance' prompted senior British microbiologist Ephraim Saul 'Andy' Anderson to warn that antimicrobial use on farms and in hospitals was leading to an uncontrolled mass-selection and spread of AMR genes. Circulating genes might accumulate in pathogens, which would then be able to resist the effects of not just one, but multiple antibiotics. He was particularly concerned about *S.* Typhi acquiring AMR genes from other *Salmonella* species, or *E. coli.*[232] This was why the 1968 Israeli article on transferable resistance in *S.* Typhi isolates was so alarming. While the Israeli strains remained sensitive to ampicillin, their detection coincided with further reports of *S.* Typhi strains with 'infective' multiple drug resistance against chloramphenicol and ampicillin from other areas in the Middle East.[225] [233] In London, Anderson feared that this was a sign of worse to come. He was right.

Starting in 1972, authorities in Mexico and the US began to detect signs of a mass outbreak of typhoid. Coming on the back of a deadly MDR *Shigella dysenteriae* outbreak, the regional typhoid outbreak, centred on Mexico City, caused over 10,000 cases, and was resistant to chloramphenicol. In parallel, new MDR typhoid outbreaks were reported from Vietnam, Korea, Thailand, India and Peru.[6]

What was driving this global surge of AMR? While it is impossible to pinpoint the exact moment when antibiotic use led to the selection and transfer of AMR in *S.* Typhi, it is possible to reconstruct the broader social and environmental factors contributing to its spread. Regardless of whether one focuses on the Mexican, Indian or Vietnamese context, there are striking similarities. During a time of global population growth and urbanisation, many citizens in all three countries lacked access to safe drinking water and effective sewage disposal. Problematic food hygiene and using sewage to irrigate crops likely further spread the disease, and public health systems were often rudimentary – particularly in rural or war-torn areas.[234]–[237] While these conditions all aided the circulation of *S.* Typhi, rising local antibiotic use was simultaneously selecting for increasingly drug-resistant strains. Although it was frequently decried as 'irrational', using cheap antibiotics to treat and prevent infections was an entirely rational response to lack of access to other health and sanitary services.[238] Over time, the combination of high local typhoid incidence and antibiotic use created ideal conditions for the rise of multiple drug-resistant *S.* Typhi strains.

Unfortunately, scientific awareness of growing AMR problems did not translate into effective action. Amidst the launch of several new effective antibiotic treatments

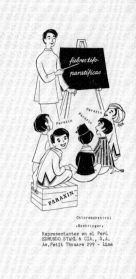

Peruvian advert promoting the use of chloramphenicol (paraxin) against typhoid and paratyphoid, Edmundo Stahl & Cia, 1958.

and two new typhoid vaccines between 1974 and 1986,* typhoid remained a neglected disease on international health agendas.[6]

SANITATION

International neglect of typhoid and AMR occurred amidst a wider revaluation of developmental investment in water and sewage systems.

Between 1972 and 1978, high-level UN initiatives such as the Stockholm, Mar Del Plata and Alma Atta conferences had led to political commitments to improve universal access to primary health care and water. The need for clean water was again emphasised during the International Decade of Water between 1981 and 1990. However, like so many other calls to action, resulting aid, credit and investment had failed to keep up with population growth and urbanisation, or to guarantee the long-term maintenance of infrastructure once it had been built.[6] [239] [240]

Politically, things were made worse by controversies about the economic cost-effectiveness of investing in sanitation and clean water. Since the Victorian era, building water and sanitary infrastructures had been seen as a crucial component of disease control and national development (Chapter 7). During the post-war years, large parts of the developmental aid community continued to believe that the benefits of water-focused investment were so self-evident that it did not need to be justified. This dogma began to be challenged during the mid-1970s. In Washington, the World Bank, under former US Secretary of Defence Robert McNamara, began to apply cost-benefit assessments to ensure that the bank's investments generated measurable value. While the impact of other technical interventions, such as vaccines, was comparatively easy to measure, economists struggled to disentangle and quantify the complex health and economic impacts of water-based interventions. Over time, econometric confusion resulted in growing hesitancy amongst international donors about investing in new water infrastructure.[226] [241]

Cost-effectiveness concerns also resulted in attempts to maximise value-generation from existing water projects in so-called developing countries. During the 1970s, many of these countries had taken out large loans to pay for industrial development and import substitution. By the 1980s, the global recession, rising interest rates and an appreciation of the US dollar meant that they now struggled to service these loans. In return for debt relief, the World Bank and International Monetary Fund insisted on the implementation of 'structural adjustment'. Although both organisations acknowledged that health was essential for economic development, their adjustment guidance followed neoliberal preferences for a 'lean state', quantifiable returns on investment and allowing market actors to take over previously public services such as water or health provision.

The 1980s and 1990s thus saw many countries, across South America, Asia and Africa, forced to decentralise, privatise and introduce user fees for essential services such as water, sewage and health. Assessing the wider societal impact of adjustment

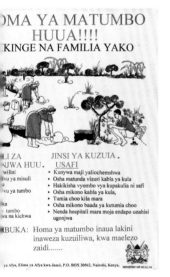

Safe water is not available everywhere. This poster created by the Kenya Ministry of Health, c.2000, warns that 'typhoid fever kills!' and informs readers about symptoms and preventative measures, including boiling water, washing fruit and using toilets. It also depicts two women using a stream, into which two men urinate and defecate.

---

* New antibiotic treatments for *S.* Typhi included trimethoprim-sulfamethoxazole (1974); first- and second-generation fluoroquinolones (norfloxacin, 1978; ofloxacin, 1980/1985; ciprofloxacin, 1987); macrolides (azithromycin, 1980/1986); and third-generation cephalosporins (ceftriaxone, 1984).

is complicated. While international relief helped states avoid defaulting on debts, commodified public services became more difficult to access for the communities that needed them most. In the case of water services, unaffordable fees for commercial supplies led the poor to rely on degraded sources, which inevitably compromised the control of typhoid and many other waterborne diseases.[226] [241] [242]

VACCINATION

Fortunately, not every field of typhoid intervention stalled. Despite waning enthusiasm for water-based interventions and lack of concern about AMR, wealthier nations continued to invest in vaccine innovation. The fact that vaccines were a limited technical intervention that could be used during health emergencies and stop the introduction of typhoid from abroad made them particularly attractive to funders.

During the Second World War, all major powers had made use of first-generation killed whole-cell typhoid vaccines and combined typhoid, paratyphoid A and B (TAB) vaccines. However, use of these vaccines in civilian populations remained limited.** Although improvements in sterilisation and the post-war introduction of disposable plastic syringes had significantly reduced the risks of cross-infection during large-scale vaccination campaigns, whole-cell vaccines triggered strong side effects, such as inflammation, pain, fever, malaise and other disease-like symptoms in up to 34 per cent of recipients, and could temporarily leave between 21 and 23 per cent of recipients unable to work. Meanwhile, production methods and the bacterial strains being used to create vaccines continued to vary.[243]

From the 1950s onwards, there was thus significant interest in evaluating the efficacy and side effects of different vaccines being produced across the world. Coordinated by the WHO, a series of large-scale field trials evaluated the efficacy of whole-cell vaccines in Yugoslavia, Poland, the USSR and British Guyana.[243] Taking a different approach, US researchers at the University of Maryland decided to test vaccine efficacy with a controlled human infection model (CHIM). Similar to the later Oxford trial (Chapter 14), the idea behind the CHIM was to first vaccinate and then infect a closely controlled target population with a live strain of *S.* Typhi. In a far cry from modern standards of informed consent, the US target population for the trial consisted of male 'volunteers' from the Maryland House of Correction[244] – a practice that was significantly curtailed between 1976 and 1978.[245] Volunteers were infected by being asked to gargle and then swallow milk that had been contaminated with the so-called Quailes strain of *S.* Typhi,[246] which had been isolated from a chronic carrier in the Maryland region.

Challenge and field trials not only highlighted the superiority of acetone-killed over alcohol- or heat-killed inactivated vaccines,[243] but also indicated ways to produce improved typhoid vaccines. Two new technologies seemed particularly promising. One approach centred on using parts or subunits of *S.* Typhi to train the

** By the 1980s, only the USSR and Thailand had launched large-scale attempts to control typhoid using whole-cell vaccines.

body's immune system. Research on the acetone (K) whole-cell vaccines had already indicated the role of *S.* Typhi's Vi-polysaccharide antigen in inducing immunity. Could injecting the Vi antigen by itself protect humans? While early challenge trials with purified Vi antigens on chimpanzees and Maryland inmates were disappointing, advances in the extraction of bacterial polysaccharides for meningococcal vaccines opened the door for a new era of subunit vaccines. Between 1972 and 1974, US researchers managed to purify *S.* Typhi's Vi antigen without denaturing it. This breakthrough led to the development of two Vi-based vaccines, by the US National Institutes of Health and the French Mérieux Institute. The commercially developed French vaccine proved to have fewer side effects, and was trialled in South Africa and Nepal, where its efficacy ranged between 64 and 72 per cent.[243]

A second approach towards vaccine innovation centred on using modified strains of *S.* Typhi to induce immunity. It had been known for some time that swallowing solutions of dead typhoid bacteria caused few adverse reactions, but did not offer protection. Could immunity without adverse effects be induced by swallowing live typhoid strains that had been rendered harmless? During the early 1970s, Swiss researchers managed to create a harmless mutant (Ty21a) strain, which lacked a Vi antigen and did not revert back to a more virulent version. When ingested, Ty21a allowed the body's immune system to learn how to recognise more virulent *S.* Typhi strains.[247] The Swiss Ty21a strains were received with great interest in the US. Supported by the Department of Defense, researchers in Maryland had already been trialling various new typhoid vaccines on 149 prison volunteers, and found that an adapted version of Ty21a offered 87 per cent protection and caused significantly fewer side effects than first-generation vaccines.[248] Further efficacy data was gathered during extensive field trials in Egypt (1978–81), Chile (1982–87) and Indonesia (1986–88).[243] While resulting data showed that oral Ty21a vaccines were safe and effective, the decision to locate all three trial sites in territories that were governed by authoritarian regimes with poor human rights records once again compromised the ability to gain meaningful informed consent from trial populations.

Despite the ethical problems surrounding their trials, the fact that second-generation subunit and mutated whole-cell vaccines were well-tolerated and effective against typhoid gave hope that a new era of vaccine-based disease control was approaching. In 1984, participants at an international workshop on typhoid noted that better diagnostics, new antimicrobials and improved vaccines 'engendered a sense of optimism … for improved, worldwide control of typhoid fever'.[249] This assessment was over-confident.

With effective monitoring of *S.* Typhi still limited to wealthy countries, there was little to no active surveillance of changing microbial dynamics, including AMR, in many high-prevalence areas. Meanwhile, few of the underlying structural factors driving the transmission of *S.* Typhi and other enteric pathogens in poorer countries had been fixed. As the next two decades would show, political and economic instability, lack or deteriorating access to clean water, crumbling health infrastructures and increasing antibiotic use would fuel a resistant surge of typhoid and threaten decades of control efforts.

Second-generation typhoid vaccines had significantly fewer side effects and could be rolled out to wider populations. This Kenyan Sanofi Pasteur poster, *c.*2000, provides information on typhoid prevention and celebrates the roll-out of Vi vaccines since 1989.

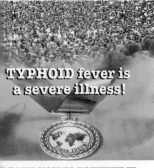

CHAPTER FOURTEEN

A perfect storm

Were a notable proportion of the enteric fever cases
in the future to become virtually untreatable because they
are caused by emergent H58 haplotype XDR strains,
this would turn the clock back to the pre-1948 era,
when typhoid fever was not treatable.

MYRON M. LEVINE AND RAPHAEL SIMON, 2018[250]

O N 12 February 2021, the American Centers for Disease Control and
Prevention (CDC) Health Alert Network carried a short warning.
Between 9 February 2018 and 16 November 2020, the agency had
received 71 reports of US cases of a new variant of extensively drug-
resistant (XDR) typhoid that was linked to an ongoing mass outbreak in Pakistan. In
58 cases, the source of infection could be linked to recent travel to the region.
However, nine patients from six states reported no history of travel, and could not be
linked to each other. Eight of these patients were hospitalised – none died. Although
the alert was overshadowed by the COVID-19 emergency, the US was experiencing a
domestic outbreak of XDR typhoid. Worryingly, the XDR strains, which were very
closely related to the ones circulating in Pakistan, proved resistant to nearly all of the
antibiotics that had been approved to treat *S*. Typhi since 1948.[251] [252]

For the many microbiologists, public health experts and international
organisations trying to tackle typhoid, the CDC Health Alert came as no great
surprise. Since the mid-1990s, they had warned about a global surge of increasingly
drug-resistant *S*. Typhi.[253] This surge had started sometime in the 1980s, and was
driven by factors such as a lack of access to safe water, sanitation and healthcare, and
due to rising antibiotic use (see Chapter 13).[6]

Initially, the surge was picked up as multiple-drug resistance (MDR) across
several *S*. Typhi phage types.[253] A fuller and more disturbing epidemiological
picture began to emerge with the establishment of genomic surveillance.
Collaborative typing of new and archived *S*. Typhi isolates with increasingly
sophisticated molecular techniques revealed that the surge of AMR was due to the
international spread of one genetically restricted clade of typhoid, which was
named haplotype 58 (H58) in 2006.[8] In the areas where it emerged, H58 displaced
other haplotypes as the dominant cause of typhoid, and was strongly associated
with multiple drug resistance.[6]

The spread of H58 coincided with increasing political and economic instability,
and the collapse of the Soviet bloc. The resulting fragility of health and water
infrastructures allowed various types of *S*. Typhi to make inroads into previously
well-controlled territories. While individual typhoid outbreaks were reported in
Eastern Europe and former Yugoslavia, the situation was particularly dire in the

newly independent republics of Central Asia. From 1996 through 1998, over 90 per cent of strains from a mass outbreak among 24,000 people in war-torn Tajikistan were multiply drug-resistant against first-line drugs and 82 per cent were resistant to the fluoroquinolone ciprofloxacin.[6]

In a vicious cycle of AMR selection, the spread of increasingly drug-resistant strains made patients abandon older first-line drugs in favour of newer antibiotics, which were being aggressively marketed and becoming more affordable.[254] This led to further selection for AMR against newer drugs. By the early 2000s, the first reports of sporadic ceftriaxone resistance began to emerge, and fluoroquinolone resistance was common across large parts of South Asia.[6] Meanwhile, the ongoing absence of effective diagnostics and laboratory infrastructure for typhoid, coupled with many patients' inability to access formal healthcare, meant that repeated appeals for 'rational' antibiotic use achieved little.[255] By 2016, the H58 strain behind Pakistan's XDR outbreak was resistant to all first-line drugs, the quinolones and ceftriaxone. Having cautioned about rising AMR for decades, the Sindh outbreak made senior microbiologists warn that the 'gathering storm' of XDR would become a 'perfect storm'[250] of untreatable typhoid if no urgent action was taken.

In Pakistan, where the outbreak had caused at least 16,000 cases by early 2020, the only antibiotics left to treat XDR typhoid were the oral macrolide azithromycin and the carbapenem meropenem. A seven- to fourteen-day course of azithromycin cost USD 5.87 per day, and could be self-administered by patients. By contrast, a similar course of meropenem cost USD 88.46 per day, and had to administered intravenously in a healthcare setting.[256] In a country where free access to these health settings was limited, and average monthly salaries range from between USD 135.03 to USD 2,380 (2021 data),[257] this difference in cost and accessibility meant that azithromycin played a vital role in keeping typhoid mortality down. Unfortunately, bacterial resistance to this popular class of macrolides seemed just around the corner. At the final plenary of the 11th international conference on typhoid in 2019, a speaker asked the audience whether anybody had observed a strain in their laboratories. Nobody answered. One year later, the detection of azithromycin-resistant S. Typhi strains was reported from Bangladesh, Pakistan and Nepal.[258]

With cases of XDR now being reported across the world, it is clear that a further loss of antibiotic efficacy will have dire consequences not just for Pakistan. As always, things will be worst for the poorest and most vulnerable with no access to safe water, sanitation and healthcare. However, as the 2021 US XDR-outbreak shows, even citizens from wealthy countries are not completely safe from resurgent typhoid in other parts of the world. For now, they can resort to effective and more expensive antibiotics. But for how long will these drugs remain effective? In the face of stalling antibiotic innovation,[259] the day may be drawing closer when a strain of S. Typhi will no longer respond to any of the antibiotics used to treat it. Because more selective evolutionary pressure is being brought to bear on fewer effective drugs, this day may come sooner than we would like to imagine.

Fortunately, there is new hope in the form of vaccination. In a remarkable parallel to the 1970s outbreaks (Chapter 13), a surge in AMR has, by chance, coincided with

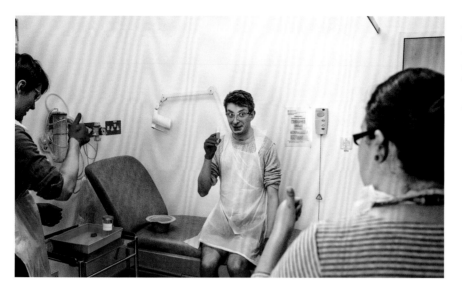

A volunteer prepares to swallow a vial of live S. Typhi during the 2017 human challenge trial of a new typhoid conjugate vaccine by the Oxford Vaccine Group.

major advances in vaccine development. During the 1990s, international organisations had already advocated the mass use of second-generation Ty21a and Vi polysaccharide vaccines to regain control of typhoid and stop the proliferation of AMR. However, despite mass roll-outs in Vietnam and China, doubts remained about typhoid vaccines' usefulness for routine disease control in endemic countries.[260] [261] The multiple doses and frequent boosters required for both vaccines made them comparatively expensive for inclusion in routine vaccine schedules. More significantly, neither vaccine offered significant protection for young children – the age group most at risk from typhoid. Vi vaccines offered less than 38 per cent protection for the two-to-five-year-old age bracket, and were not effective below two years of age. Meanwhile, Ty21a capsules could only be safely administered to children above five years of age. These limitations also meant that second-generation typhoid vaccines were deemed unsuitable for support by GAVI, the global vaccine alliance, which had been founded in 2000 and was fast becoming a vital source of financial support when it came to vaccine roll-outs in poorer countries.[262]–[264]

What was needed was a new generation of vaccines that would protect the youngest and most vulnerable in areas without adequate sanitation, and ideally require just one dose. By the early 2000s, multiple promising vaccines were already in development. One group of candidates consisted of live attenuated vaccines with novel mutations, which would render S. Typhi harmless and induce immunity after oral ingestion.[264] Another group of vaccines used the principle of conjugation to overcome the limits of existing typhoid vaccines. First conceived of during the late 1980s, conjugate vaccines fuse – or conjugate – the purified polysaccharide (antigen) of a pathogen with another substance that provides a strong and lasting immune memory. In most cases, this second substance is a toxoid protein (from diphtheria or tetanus), which is easily recognised by the immune system. During the 1990s, conjugate vaccines against *Haemophilus influenzae* type B (HiB), *Pneumococcus* and various serogroups of *Meningococcus* had already been licensed.[265]

Relying on a mix of for-profit and non-profit capital, multiple companies also began to develop so-called Vi conjugate vaccines that were based on conjugating the

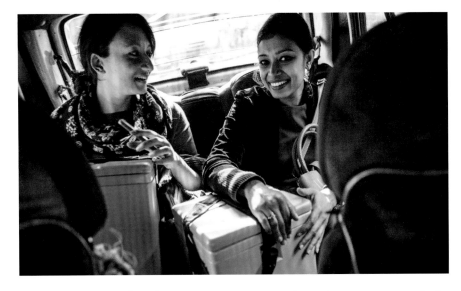

Bringing the new TCV vaccine to Nepalese trial sites in cool bags.

purified Vi polysaccharide to carrier proteins such as the tetanus toxoid, the diphtheria toxoid (CRM) and the recombinant ExoProtein A of *Pseudomonas aeruginosa* (rEPA). The road to licensing was long and stony. Published in 1999, a rEPA-based conjugate vaccine by French company Pasteur Mérieux Connaught showed promising results across age groups in early-stage trials in Vietnam, but only progressed slowly through subsequent trials.[266] In 2011, the Siena-based Novartis Global Health Institute reported promising trials of a new conjugate vaccine employing a non-toxic mutant of the diphtheria toxin (Vi-CRM197).[263] An additional conjugate vaccine based on a diphtheria toxoid carrier protein (Vi-DT) was developed by the International Vaccine Institute in Korea, and began to be trialled in the Philippines in 2016.[267]

However, it was in India that the race to license the first typhoid conjugate vaccines was won. Around 2010, the two biotech companies Bharat Biotech and Bio-Med each began testing tetanus toxoid-based conjugate vaccines. While Bio-Med's Peda-Typh vaccine was licensed in India by 2011,[268] [269]★ Bharat Biotech's Typbar TCV was the first to gain international approval. Following an Indian phase three trial between 2011 and 2012, the 2017 Oxford human challenge trial results provided sufficient evidence of safety and immunogenicity for Typbar TCV to receive WHO prequalification and the all-important GAVI support in 2018. Further large-scale trials in Nepal and India were subsequently conducted to gather data on implementation and galvanise international support.[268] [270]

The ability of the Bharat TCV to induce around 82 per cent protection against typhoid in children as young as six months old after one dose was heralded as a game-changer.[213] [270] It also led to the mass roll-out of the vaccine to over ten million school children in Pakistan in late 2019 in an attempt to control the Sindh Province XDR-outbreak and TCV's subsequent adoption in other countries.[271] To most observers, it seemed as though conjugate vaccines had opened up new and affordable vistas for typhoid control beyond wealthy nations' borders.

★ At the time of licensing in India, Bio-Med had not published full efficacy and trial data.

CHAPTER FIFTEEN

Conclusion:
Taking typhoid seriously

OUR KNOWLEDGE OF TYPHOID FEVER has come a long way since Pierre-Charles-Alexandre Louis coined the term almost two hundred years ago. Some 126 years after the first whole-cell typhoid vaccines were trialled on humans, there are now two WHO-prequalified typhoid conjugate vaccines (TCV) that do not cause significant side effects, are effective in all age groups and require only one shot. Meanwhile, at least three further promising TCVs are in various stages of development – with calls growing to create a combined bivalent vaccine for typhoid and paratyphoid.[272] The salient question is whether these new vaccines will be enough to overcome decades of international neglect of typhoid and calm the gathering storm of XDR.

Looking back at the last two centuries of typhoid control efforts, the answer is: not by themselves. In contrast to the booster rhetoric that surrounded the initial TCV roll-out in Pakistan, follow-up surveys by social scientists are showing that vaccine advocacy and uptake among many frontline healthcare workers remain comparatively low, and that non-targeted antibiotic use against suspected typhoid remains common.[273]

These findings should not surprise us. Historically, effective vaccine campaigns have almost never been a substitute for other forms of disease control, but have only ever worked as a complement to broader public health and sanitary interventions. Similar to the roll-out of first-generation typhoid vaccines around 1900 and the licensing of second-generation vaccines during the 1980s, TCVs' long-term impact on typhoid will depend just as much on their biological efficacy as on the wider social and environmental context of their adoption.

Key to any TCV success will be to engage in continuous vaccine advocacy among local communities, guarantee the long-term financial and physical accessibility of vaccines and simultaneously create sustainable laboratory, water and health infrastructures to control typhoid in different geographic contexts. The basic toolkit for controlling typhoid has existed since the early twentieth century. However, as this book has shown, expert knowledge of disease dynamics and effective interventions is not the same as implementing a successful programme of long-term control. On the ground, public health is inevitably messy. Populations do not necessarily comply with what planners think is 'rational', local elites may have competing agendas, and disease and hydrological environments may be very different from those in public health textbooks. All of this means that achieving meaningful progress towards typhoid control will be difficult, and that effective solutions will likely vary across regional contexts.

What is needed in order to achieve these solutions is a system of international support that is both flexible enough to respond to local concerns and robust enough to provide the long-term financial and logistical backing for a progressive optimisation and adaptation of control measures – not just over years but over decades. At the international level, creating such a system will entail revising some of the post-1970s cost-effectiveness approaches that have often facilitated the prioritisation of quantifiable technical short-term interventions over long-term structural support of broader health and water infrastructures. Crucially, it will also entail cultural work both for the acceptance of interventions among target populations and for the necessity of international solidarity among wealthier nations. Challenging the flawed narrative of typhoid as a disease of the past is a necessary first step.

As this book has shown, typhoid has accompanied humanity for millennia. Seen from this perspective, the relative respite that populations in wealthy nations have enjoyed from *S. Typhi* has been brief. In contrast to popular histories of a great 'sanitary awakening' and scientific breakthroughs, effective disease control depended just as much on societies' ability to mobilise resources to reshape hydrological environments, produce safe food, create accessible health services and finance biomedical innovation. The wealth and research that underpinned these achievements resulted both from economic prowess and an often-extractive global economic and political order that redirected resources from poorer to richer parts of the world. While none of this distracts from the significant achievements of early typhoid control, it should make us wary of the triumphalism that facilitated decades of international neglect of typhoid in poorer countries. This lack of collective responsibility has carried a high cost in human lives, and may yet come back to haunt inhabitants of richer countries in the form of untreatable strains of *S. Typhi*. One can only hope that the shared global tragedy of COVID-19 will create greater understanding, compassion and support for the many regions of the world where the ancient disease of typhoid remains a potent menace.

Children holding up inked fingers to show that they have been vaccinated amidst a 2021 WHO-supported Pakistani mass immunisation campaign against typhoid with the TCV vaccine.

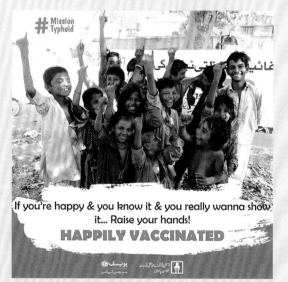

1   M.A. Evans (George Eliot), Middlemarch (London: William Blackwood and Sons, 1871/72).

2   R. Wall, Bacteria in Britain, 1880–1939 (London: Routledge, 2014).

3   J. Steere-Williams, The Filth Disease: Typhoid Fever and the Practices of Epidemiology in Victorian England (Rochester: University of Rochester Press, 2020).

4   A. Hardy, Salmonella Infections. Networks of Knowledge, and Public Health in Britain. 1880–1975 (Oxford: Oxford University Press, 2014).

5   WHO Typhoid Key Facts (31.01.2018) [accessed: 20.10.2021].

6   C. Kirchhelle, Z. A. Dyson and G. Dougan, 'A Biohistorical Perspective of Typhoid and Antimicrobial Resistance,' Clinical Infectious Diseases 69 Suppl. 5 (2019), S388–94.

7   For more information, see: www.typhoidland.org.

8   P. Roumagnac et al., 'Evolutionary history of Salmonella Typhi,' Science 314/5803 (2006), 1301–04.

9   V.K. Wong et al., 'An extended genotyping framework for Salmonella enterica serovar Typhi, the cause of human typhoid,' Nature Communications 7/1 (2016).

10   J. Worley et al., 'Salmonella enterica phylogeny based on whole-genome sequencing reveals two new clades and novel patterns of horizontally acquired genetic elements,' mBio 9/6 (2018).

11   O. Gal-Mor, 'Persistent infection and long-term carriage of typhoidal and nontyphoidal salmonellae,' Clinical Microbiology Reviews 32/1 (2019).

12   V.K. Wong et al., 'Phylogeographical analysis of the dominant multidrug-resistant H58 clade of Salmonella Typhi identifies inter- and intracontinental transmission events,' Nature Genetics 47/6 (2015), 632–39.

13   M.J. Blaser and L.S. Newman, 'A Review of Human Salmonellosis. Infective Dose,' Reviews of Infectious Diseases 4/6 (1982), 1096–1106.

14   J. V. Ashurst, J. Truong and B. Woodbury, Salmonella Typhi (Florida: Statpearls Publishing, 2021).

15   B. Basnyat et al., 'Enteric fever,' BMJ 372 (2021), n437.

16   'Cholera Illness and Symptoms,' CDC [accessed: 10.08.2021].

17   R. Adler and E. Mara, Typhoid fever: A history (Jefferson: Mcfarland & Company, 2016).

18   J. Pickstone, 'Bureaucracy, liberalism and the body in post-revolutionary France: Bichat's physiology and the Paris school of medicine,' History of Science 19/2 (1981), 115–42.

19   E.R. Müllener, 'Pierre-Charles-Alexandre Louis' (1787–1872). Genfer Schüler und die 'méthode numérique',' Gesnerus 24/1-2 (1967), 46–74.

20   A. Morabia, 'Pierre-Charles-Alexandre Louis and the evaluation of bloodletting,' Journal of the Royal Society of Medicine 99/3 (2006), 158–60.

21   D.C. Smith, 'Gerhard's distinction between typhoid and typhus and its reception in America, 1833–1860,' Bulletin of the History of Medicine 54/3 (1980), 368–85.

22   P.-C.-A. Louis, Recherches Anatomiques, Pathologiques Et Thérapeutiques sur la Maladie Connue Sous les Noms de Gastro-entérite, Fièvre Putride, Adynamique, Ataxique, Typhoïde, Etc. 2 vols (Paris: J.-B. Baillière, 1829).

23   M. Pelling, Cholera fever and English medicine (Oxford: Oxford University Press, 1978).

24   W. Jenner, 'On typhoid and typhus fevers,' Monthly Journal of Medical Science 3/38, 40, 42 (1849).

25   W. Schupbach, 'The last moments of HRH the Prince Consort,' Medical History 26/3 (1982), 321–24.

26   Queen Victoria's account of the Prince Consort's illness and death (14.12.1861 – written Feb 1872), Prince Albert's Family Papers (RA VIC/MAIN/Z/142).

27   R. English, 'Was Albert killed by Crohn's disease? Prince's death has been blamed on typhoid until now,' Daily Mail, 2011.

28   J.W. Paulley, 'The Death of Albert Prince Consort: the case against typhoid fever,' QJM 86/12 (1993), 837–41.

29   W. Budd, 'On the Fever at the Clergy Orphan Asylum,' Lancet 68/1736 (1856), 617–19.

30   T. Koch, Disease Maps. Epidemics On The Ground (Chicago: University of Chicago Press, 2011).

31   M. Harrison, Disease and the Modern World: 1500 to the Present Day (Cambridge: Polity Press, 2004).

32   F. Jarrige and T. le Roux, 'Naissance de l'enquête: les hygiénistes, Villermé et les ouvriers autour de 1840,' in É Geerkens et al. (eds) Les enquêtes ouvrières dans l'Europe contemporaine (Paris: La Découverte, 2019), 39–52.

33   A. Hardy, The epidemic streets: infectious disease and the rise of preventive medicine, 1856–1900 (Oxford: Clarendon Press, 1993).

34   J. Downs, Maladies of Empire: How Colonialism, Slavery, and War Transformed Medicine. (Boston: Harvard University Press, 2021).

35   C. Hamlin, Public Health and Social Justice in the Age of Chadwick: Britain, 1800–1854 (Cambridge: Cambridge University Press, 1998).

36   S.P.W. Chave, 'Henry Whitehead and cholera in Broad Street,' Medical History 2/2 (1958), 92–108.

37   M. Pelling, 'Mythological endings: John Snow (1813–1858) and the history of American epidemiology,' Centaurus 3 (2022).

38   R. Moorhead, 'William Budd and typhoid fever,' Journal of the Royal Society of Medicine 95/11 (2002), 561–64.

39   W. Budd, 'Mode of Propagation of Cholera,' Lancet 67/1701 (1856), 379.

40   C.J. Eberth, 'Die Organismen in den Organen by Typhus abdominalis,' Archiv für pathologische Anatomie und Physiologie und für klinische Medizin 81 (1880), 58–74.

41   C. Gradmann, Krankheit im Labor. Robert Koch und die medizinische Bakteriologie (Göttingen: Wallstein, 2005).

42   C. Gradmann, '"A Spirit of Scientific Rigour": Koch's Postulates and 20th Century Medicine,' Microbes and Infection 16/11 (2014), 885–92.

43   R. Koch, 'Zur Untersuchung von pathogenen Organismen,' Mittheilungen aus dem kaiserlichen Gesundheitsamte 1 (1881), 1–48.

44   G. Gaffky, 'Zur Aetiologie des Abdominaltyphus,' *Mittheilungen aus dem kaiserlichen Gesundheitsamte* 2 (1884), 372–403.

45   F. Widal, 'On The Sero–Diagnosis of Typhoid Fever,' *Lancet* 148/3820 (1896), 1371–72.

46   M.García, 'Typhoid fever in nineteenth-century Colombia: Between medical geography and bacteriology,' *Medical History* 58/1 (2014), 27–45.

47   I.N. Okeke, *Divining without seeds: The case for strengthening laboratory medicine in Africa* (Ithaka: Cornell University Press, 2011).

48   J.S. Haller, 'Medical thermometry – A short history,' *Western Journal of Medicine* 142/1 (1985), 108–16.

49   W.D. Forster, *A History of Medical Bacteriology and Immunology* (London: Heinemann, 1970).

50   S. Gordon, 'Elie Metchnikoff: Father of natural immunity,' *European Journal of Immunology* 38/12 (2008), 3257–64.

51   D.D. Chaplin, 'Overview of the immune response,' *Journal of Allergy and Clinical Immunology* 125/2 (Supp. 2) (2010).

52   W.E. Paul, *Immunity* (Baltimore: Johns Hopkins University Press, 2015).

53   A. Grafe, *A History of Experimental Virology* (Berlin/Heidelberg: Springer, 1991).

54   A. Charin and C.–H. Roger, 'Action du serum des animaux malades ou vaccines sur les microbes pathogenes,' *C R Scéances Acad Sci Serie D* 109 (1889), 710–13.

55   A.C. Hüntelmann, 'Evaluation as a Practical Technique of Administration: The Regulation and Standardization of Diphtheria Serum,' in C. Gradmann and J. Simon (eds), *Evaluating and Standardizing Therapeutic Agents, 1890–1950* (New York and Basingstoke: Palgrave Macmillan, 2010), 31–51.

56   A. Hardy, 'From Diphtheria to Tetanus: The Development of Evaluation Methods for Sera,' in C. Gradmann and J. Simon (eds.), *Evaluating and Standardizing Therapeutic Agents, 1890–1950* (New York and Basingstoke: Palgrave Macmillan, 2010), 52–70.

57   P.R. Hunter, 'Fernand Widal,' *Medical History* 7/1 (1963), 56–61.

58   E.T. Fison, 'Widal's Sero-Diagnosis of Typhoid Fever,' *BMJ* 2/1909 (1897), 266–69.

59   J.S.K. Boyd, 'Laboratory Methods in the Diagnosis and Control of Fevers of the Enteric Group,' *BMJ* 2/4113 (1939), 902–04.

60   O. Ajibola et al., 'Typhoid Fever Diagnosis in Endemic Countries: A Clog in the Wheel of Progress?,' *Medicina* 54/2 (2018).

61   R.G. Mather et al., 'Redefining typhoid diagnosis: what would an improved test need to look like?' *BMJ Global Health* 4/5 (2019), e001831.

62   C.E.A. Winslow, *The evolution and significance of the modern public health campaign* (New Haven: Yale University Press, 1923).

63   'Typhoid Fever at Oxford,' *Lancet* 105/2679 (1875), 28–29.

64   J.L.A. Webb Jr, *The Guts of the Matter: A Global History of Human Waste and Infectious Intestinal Disease* (Cambridge: Cambridge University Press, 2019).

65   E. Chance et al. *A History of the County of Oxford: Volume 4, the City of Oxford*. Edited by A. Crossley and C.R. Elrington (London: Victoria County History, 1979) [accessed: 22.06.2021].

66   J. Parfit, *The health of a city: Oxford, 1770–1974* (Oxford: Amate Press, 1987).

67   S. Burt and T. Burt, *Oxford Weather and Climate since 1767* (Oxford: Oxford University Press, 2019).

68   S. Jenkins, 'Floods in Oxford,' *Oxford History – Floods*, [accessed: 14.08.2021].

69   *A Report Of The Evidence Taken Before T. MacDougal Smith Into The State Of The Sewerage, Drainage, And Water Supply Of the University And City of Oxford* (Oxford: J. Vincent, 1851).

70   Health of Towns Association, *Report of the Sub-Committee on the answers returned to questions addressed to the principal towns of England and Wales, and on the objections from corporate bodies to the Public Health Bill* (London: W. Clowes and Sons, 1848).

71   H.H. Crawley, 'The history of Oxford's water supply 1615–1946,' *J British Water Works Assoc* XXIX (1947), 89–106.

72   H.L. Thompson, *Henry George Liddell D.D., Dean of Christ Church, Oxford – A Memoir* (London: John Murray, 1899).

73   H.W. Acland, *Memoir on the cholera at Oxford, in the year 1854, with considerations suggested by the epidemic* (London: J. Churchill etc., 1856).

74   J.B. Atlay, *Sir Henry Wentworth Acland – A Memoir* (London: Smith, Elder & Co., 1903).

75   W.R. Ormerod, *On the sanatory condition of Oxford* (Oxford: Ashmolean Society, 1848).

76   W.A. Greenhill, *Report on the mortality and public health of Oxford during the years 1849, 1850* (Oxford: Ashmolean Society, 1850).

77   R.J. Morris, 'Religion and medicine: the cholera pamphlets of Oxford, 1832, 1849 and 1854,' *Medical History* 19/3 (1975), 256–70.

78   S. Vanderslott et al., 'Water and Filth: Reevaluating the First Era of Sanitary Typhoid Intervention (1840–1940),' *Clinical Infectious Diseases* 69 Suppl. 5 (2019), S377–84.

79   G.W. Child, *The Removal of Iffley Lock considered in relation to the Health of Oxford* (Oxford: Slatter and Rose, 1885).

80   R.C. Whiting, *Oxford: Studies in the History of a University Town Since 1800* (Manchester: Manchester University Press, 1993).

81   'Drainage of the Oxford Valley Scheme,' *Lancet* 127/3268 (1886), 753.

82   'Report of the Lancet Sanitary Commission on Drainage of Eton and Windsor Castle,' *Lancet* 104/2668 (1874), 564.

83   'Typhoid fever at Oxford,' *Lancet* 104/2677 (1874), 883.

84   'Annus Medicus,' *Lancet* 104/2678 (1874), 910.

85   'Annotations,' *Lancet* 105/2703 (1875), 873.

86   'The Illness of Prince Leopold,' *New York Times* (07.02.1875), 9.

87   B. Harris and A. Hinde, 'Sanitary investment and the decline of urban mortality in England and Wales, 1817–1914,' *The History of the Family* 24/2 (2019), 339–76.

88   'Contagious Diseases Act,' *Lancet* 97/2475 (1871), 169.

89   J.C. Riddell, 'Modern Methods of Sewage Disposal,' *Journal of the Royal Society of Health* 78/3 (1958), 285–92.

90   A. Carpenter, 'Utilisation Of Town Sewage By Irrigation,' *Journal of the Society of Arts* 35 (1886), 221–40.

91   'A Medical Officer of Health For Oxford,' *Lancet* 98/2520 (1871), 861.

92   'Sewage Grass and Typhoid Fever,' *Jackson's Oxford Journal* (30.08.1873).

93   G.A. Rowell, 'On the Surface Ventilation of the Public Sewers and the Cause of Cholera,' *Jackson's Oxford Journal* (23.08.1884).

94   'Sanitary Notes and Reports,' *Lancet* 106/2713 (1875), 326.

95   'The Oxford Drainage Scheme,' *Jackson's Oxford Journal* (03.05.1873).

96   'Drainage At Oxford,' *Lancet* 103/2629 (1874), 101.

97   Acland Consultation on Littlemore Asylum, 29.04.1874, MS Acland d3, Acland Papers, Weston Library, University of Oxford.

98 'Report of the Lancet Sanitary Commission on the drainage and general sanitary condition in Oxford,' *Lancet* 104/2673 (1874), 742–44.

99 'Radcliffe Infirmary,' *Jackson's Oxford Journal* (04.12.1875).

100 G.A. Rowell, 'The Drainage of Oxford and the Watercloset System,' *Jackson's Oxford Journal* (13.01.1872).

101 'Oxford Local Board,' *Jackson's Oxford Journal* (27.01.1872).

102 G. Rolleston, 'Typhoid Or Enteric Fever in Indian Gaols, and on the relations of that disease and of cholera to the dry-earth system of conservancy,' *Lancet* 94/2471 (1871), 7.

103 'Professor Rolleston on the Dry Earth System of Conservancy,' *Lancet* 97/2474 (1871), 141.

104 'Untitled,' *Lancet* 118/3026 (1881), 394.

105 'Annus Medicus, 1875,' *Lancet* 106/2730 (1875), 921.

106 F. Bell and R. Millward, 'Public health expenditures and mortality in England and Wales 1870–1914,' *Continuity and Change* 13/2 (1998), 221–49.

107 'Licensed Lodgings At Oxford,' *Lancet* 118/3024 (1881), 295.

108 'The Typhoid Epidemic at Maidstone,' *Journal of the Sanitary Institute* 18/3 (1897), 388.

109 *White's Handbook of chlorination and alternative disinfectants* [5th edition] (New York: John Wiley and Sons, 2010).

110 R. Stanwell-Smith, 'The Maidstone typhoid outbreak of 1897: an important centenary,' *Weekly releases* 1/29 (1997), 1027.

111 D. Schoenen, 'Role of disinfection in suppressing the spread of pathogens with drinking water: possibilities and limitations,' *Water Research* 36/15 (2002), 3874–88.

112 M.J. McGuire, *The chlorine revolution: water disinfection and the fight to save lives* (Denver: American Water Works Association, 2013).

113 'Typhoid Fever At Cambridge,' *Lancet* 103/2633 (1874), 240.

114 'The Sanitary Condition Of Our Universities,' *Lancet* 105/2688 (1875), 353.

115 'Licensed Lodging Houses at Oxford,' *Lancet* 119/3065 (1882), 879.

116 Oxford Local Board, *Medical Officer's Report for 1887* (Oxford: Chronicle Company, 1888), 9.

117 'The Critical Faculty in Medical Officers of Health,' *Lancet* 106/2730 (1875), 926.

118 Joseph Lister to Henry Acland, 16.12.1891, MS Acland, d. 64, Acland Papers, Weston Library, University of Oxford.

119 E. Webster, *Microbial Empires: Changing Ecologies and Multispecies Epidemics in British Imperial Cities, 1837–1910* (University of Chicago: PhD Dissertation, 2021).

120 H.A. Roechling, 'The Sewage-farms of Berlin,' *Minutes of the Proceedings of the Institution of Civil Engineers* 109 (1892), 179–228.

121 J.S. Gauld et al, 'Typhoid fever in Santiago, Chile: Insights from a mathematical model utilizing venerable archived data from a successful disease control program,' *PLOS Neglected Tropical Diseases* 12/9 (2018), e0006759.

122 F.W. Tanner, 'Public health significance of sewage sludge when used as a fertilizer,' *Sewage Works Journal* (1935), 611–17.

123 G.M. Doreen et al., 'Investigation of the fate of sulfonamides downgradient of a decommissioned sewage farm near Berlin, Germany,' *Journal of contaminant hydrology* 106/3-4 (2009), 183–94.

124 H. Ritchie, 'The world is making progress on clean water and sanitation, but is far behind its target to ensure universal access by 2030,' *Our World in Data*, 01.07.2021 [accessed: 17.01.2022].

125 C.A. Cameron, 'On Sewage in Oysters,' *BMJ* 2/1029 (1880): 471.

126 V.J. Cirillo, '"Winged Sponges": Houseflies as Carriers of Typhoid Fever in 19th- and Early 20th-Century Military Camps,' *Perspectives in Biology and Medicine* 49/1 (2006), 52–63.

127 N. Tomes, *The gospel of germs: men, women, and the microbe in American life* (Harvard: Harvard University Press, 1998).

128 A. Hardy, 'Exorcizing Molly Malone: Typhoid and Shellfish Consumption in Urban Britain 1860–1960,' *History Workshop Journal* 55/1 (2003), 72–90.

129 A. Hardy, 'Salad Days: The Science and Medicine of Bad Greens, 1870–2000,' in A.N.H. Creager and J.-P. Gaudillière (eds), *Risk on the table: food production, health, and the environment* (New York and Oxford: Berghahn, 2021), 29–54.

130 R. Ford, 'Controlling contagion? Watercress, regulation and the Hackney typhoid outbreak of 1903,' *Rural History* 31/2 (2020), 181–94.

131 C.O. Melick, 'The Possibility of Typhoid Infection Through Vegetables,' *Journal of Infectious Diseases* 21/1 (1917), 28–38.

132 A. Ceredi, 'Green Vegetables in the Epidemiology of Typhoid Fever,' *Igiene Moderna* 7/1 (1929).

133 K. Smith-Howard, *Pure and modern milk: an environmental history since 1900* (Oxford: Oxford University Press, 2013).

134 J. Steere-Williams, 'The perfect food and the filth disease: milk-borne typhoid and epidemiological practice in late Victorian Britain,' *Journal of the history of medicine and allied sciences* 65/4 (2010), 514–45.

135 L.G. Wilson, 'The historical riddle of milk-borne scarlet fever,' *Bulletin of the History of Medicine* 60/3 (1986), 321–42.

136 W.R. Stokes and H.W. Stoner, 'Isolation of the typhoid bacillus from milk which caused a typhoid outbreak,' *JAMA* 61/13 part 1 (1913), 1024–27.

137 J.F. Anderson, 'The Frequency of Tubercle Bacilli in the Market Milk of the City of Washington, D.C.,' *Journal of Infectious Diseases* 5/2 (1908), 107–15.

138 K. Waddington, *The bovine scourge: meat, tuberculosis and public health, 1850–1914* (Woodbridge: Boydell & Brewer, 2006).

139 D.G. Pritchard, 'A century of bovine tuberculosis 1888–1988: conquest and controversy,' *Journal of comparative pathology* 99/4 (1988), 357–99.

140 R.W. Currier and J.A. Widness, 'A Brief History of Milk Hygiene and Its Impact on Infant Mortality from 1875 to 1925 and Implications for Today,' *Journal of food protection* 81/10 (2018), 1713–22.

141 P.J. Atkins, 'The pasteurisation of England: the science, culture and health implications of milk processing, 1900–1950,' in D.F. Smith and J. Phikips (eds.), *Food, Science, Policy and Regulation in the Twentieth Century* (London and New York: Routledge, 1999), 37–51.

142 S. Berger, *Bakterien in Krieg und Frieden: Eine Geschichte der medizinischen Bakteriologie in Deutschland, 1890–1933* (Göttingen: Wallstein Verlag, 2009).

143 M. Worboys, 'Was there a Bacteriological Revolution in late nineteenth-century medicine?' *Studies in History and Philosophy of Science Part C* 38/1 (2007), 20–42.

144 'Oysters and Disease,' *The Times* (01.12.1896).

145 R. Koch, 'Die Bekämpfung des Typhus,' Vortrag, gehalten in der Sitzung des Wissenschaftlichen Senats bei der Kaiser-Wilhelms-Akademie am 28. November 1902 (Berlin: Hirschwald, 1903) – author's translation.

146 United States Surgeon-General's Office, *Abstract of report on the origin and spread of typhoid fever in US military camps during the Spanish war of 1898* (Washington DC: GPO, 1900).

147   V.J. Cirillo, 'Fever and reform: the typhoid epidemic in the Spanish-American War,' *Journal of the history of medicine and allied sciences* 55/4 (2000), 363–97.

148   C. Gradmann, 'Robert Koch and the Invention of the Carrier State: Tropical Medicine, Veterinary Infections and Epidemiology around 1900,' *Studies in History and Philosophy of Biological and Biomedical Sciences* 41/3 (2010), 232–40.

149   C. Gradmann, M. Harrison and A. Rasmussen, 'Typhoid and the Military in the Early 20th Century,' *Clinical Infectious Diseases* 69 Suppl. 5 (2019), S385–87.

150   A.J. Mendelsohn, *Cultures of Bacteriology: Formation and Transformation of a Science in France and Germany, 1870–1914.* (Princeton: PhD Dissertation, 1996).

151   M. Hammerborg, 'The Campaign to Eradicate Typhoid Fever in Western Norway,' in A. Andresen et al. (eds)., *Healthcare Systems and Medical Institutions* (Oslo: Novus, 2009), 170–85.

152   P.P. Mortimer, 'Mr N the milker, and Dr Koch's concept of the healthy carrier,' *Lancet* 353/9161 (1999), 1354–56.

153   A.M. Kraut, *Silent travelers: germs, genes, and the 'immigrant menace'* (Baltimore: Johns Hopkins University Press, 1995).

154   S. Trubeta, C. Promitzer, and P. Weindling (eds), *Medicalising borders: selection, containment and quarantine since 1800* (Manchester: Manchester University Press, 2021).

155   J. Walzer Leavitt, *Typhoid Mary: captive to the public's health* (Boston: Beacon Press, 1996).

156   C. Hooker, 'Sanitary failure and risk: pasteurisation, immunisation and the logics of prevention,' in A. Bashford and C. Hooker (eds), *Contagion. Historical and cultural studies* (London and New York: Routledge, 2001), 129–52.

157   W. Anderson, 'Excremental Colonialism: Public Health and the Poetics of Pollution,' *Critical Inquiry* 21/3 (1995), 640–69.

158   B.E. Crim, '"Our Most Serious Enemy": The Specter of Judeo-Bolshevism in the German Military Community, 1914–1923,' *Central European History* 44/4 (2011), 624–41.

159   'Typhoid women were kept in asylum,' BBC (28.07.2008) [accessed: 16.08.2021].

160   Vere Knight, 'City Volunteers,' *Jackson's Oxford Journal* (17.03.1900).

161   P.J. Marshall, ed., *The Cambridge illustrated history of the British Empire* (Cambridge: Cambridge University Press, 2001).

162   'Imperial Yeomanry,' *Jackson's Oxford Journal* (03.03.1900).

163   W.H. Crumley, 'Letters from the front,' *Jackson's Oxford Journal* (05.05.1900).

164   V. Knight, 'City Volunteers,' *Jackson's Oxford Journal* (17.03.1900).

165   'Spoiling Our Soldiers,' *Jackson's Oxford Journal* (06.01.1900).

166   C. Brake, 'What Verdict On Typhoid Inoculation,' *Jackson's Oxford Journal* (02.06.1900).

167   S. Blume, *Immunization: How Vaccines became Controversial* (London: Reaktion Books, 2017).

168   J.D. Williamson, K.G. Gould and K. Brown, 'Richard Pfeiffer's typhoid vaccine and Almroth Wright's claim to priority,' *Vaccine* 39/15 (2021), 2074–79.

169   P.G. Fildes, 'Richard Friedrich Johannes Pfeiffer, 1858–1945,' *Biogr. Mems Fell. R. Soc.* 2 (1956), 237–47.

170   D.H.M. Groschel and R.B.Hornick, 'Who Introduced Typhoid Vaccination: Almroth Wright or Richard Pfeiffer?' *Review of Infectious Diseases* 3/6 (1981), 1251–54.

171   G.H. Bornside, 'Waldemar Haffkine's cholera vaccines and the Ferran-Haffkine priority dispute,' *Journal of the history of medicine and allied sciences* 37/4 (1982), 399–422.

172   R. Pfeiffer and W. Kolle, 'Experimentelle Untersuchungen zur Frage der Schutzimpfung des Menschen gegen typhus abdominalis,' *DMW* 22/46 (1896), 735–37.

173   A. Wright, 'On the association of serious haemorrhages with conditions of defective blood-coagulability,' *Lancet* 148/3812 (1896), 807–09.

174   M. Worboys, 'Almroth Wright at Netley: modern medicine and the military in Britain, 1892–1902,' in R. Cooter, M. Harrison and S. Sturdy (eds), *Medicine and modern warfare* (Leiden: Brill, 1999), 77–97.

175   A.E. Wright and D. Semple, 'Remarks on vaccination against typhoid fever,' *BMJ* 1/1883 (1897), 256–59.

176   A. Hardy, '"Straight back to barbarism": antityphoid inoculation and the Great War, 1914,' *Bulletin of the History of Medicine* 74/2 (2000), 265–90.

177   C.A. Mense, *Handbuch der Tropenkrankheiten. Zweiter Band* (Leipzig: Johann Ambrosius Barth, 1905).

178   H. Cayley, 'A Note on the Value of Inoculation Against Enteric Fever,' *BMJ* 1/2089 (1901), 84.

179   V.J. Cirillo, 'Arthur Conan Doyle (1859–1930): physician during the typhoid epidemic in the Anglo-Boer War (1899–1902),' *Journal of medical biography* 22/1 (2014), 2–8.

180   F.P. Gay, *Typhoid fever considered as a problem of scientific medicine* (New York: MacMillan, 1918).

181   W.D. Tigertt, 'The initial effort to immunize American soldier volunteers with typhoid vaccine,' *Military Medicine* 124/5 (1959), 342–49.

182   J.S. Siler, *The Medical Department of the United States Army in the World War. Vol. IX: Communicable And Other Diseases* (Washington DC: GPO, 1928).

183   G.R. Callender and G.F. Luippold, 'The effectiveness of typhoid vaccine prepared by the US Army,' *JAMA* 123/6 (1943), 319–21.

184   B. Wintermute, *Public Health and the US Military: a history of the Army Medical Department, 1818–1917* (London and New York: Routledge, 2011).

185   P. Osten, 'Militärmedizin: Unvorbereitet in die Krise,' *Deutsches Ärzteblatt* 112/9 (2015), 370–72.

186   N.T. Karasek, *Seuchen und Militär 1914–1918* (MA Dissertation: Universität Wien, 2012).

187   M. Thiessen, *Immunisierte Gesellschaft. Impfen in Deutschland im 19. und 20. Jahrhundert* (Göttingen: Vandenhoeck & Rupprecht, 2017).

188   M. Scharf, 'Im Kampf gegen den "inneren Feind",' *Habsburger.net.* [accessed: 17.08.2021].

189   S.L. Hoch, 'The social consequences of Soviet immunization policies, 1945–1980,' *National Council for Eurasian and East European Research* (1997) [accessed: 19.08.2021].

190   W. Coleman, 'Diet in Typhoid Fever,' *JAMA* LIII/15 (1909), 1145–50.

191   L.F. Barker, 'The Diet in Typhoid Fever,' *JAMA* LXIII/11 (1914), 929–31.

192   W.F. Schoffman, 'Banana diet in the treatment of typhoid fever in children: Preliminary report,' *Journal of Paediatrics* 18/3 (1941), 399–404.

193 J.T.C. Nash, 'The Diet of Typhoid Fever,' BMJ 2/2346 (1905), 1616.

194 J.R. McTavish, 'Antipyretic Treatment and Typhoid Fever: 1860–1900,' Journal of the History of Medicine and Allied Sciences 42/4 (1987), 486–506.

195 W.H. Riley, 'The Treatment of Typhoid Fever Without Alcohol,' JAMA XXV/12 (1895), 489–90.

196 M.W. Richardson, 'On the Value of Urotropin as a Urinary Antiseptic with Especial Reference to Its Use in Typhoid Fever,' Journal of Experimental Medicine 4/1 (1899), 19.

197 R.D. Roy, Malarial Subjects: Empire, Medicine and Nonhumans in British India, 1820–1909 (Cambridge: Cambridge University Press, 2017).

198 G. Dutfield, That High Design of Purest Gold: A Critical History of the Pharmaceutical Industry, 1880–2020 (Singapore: World Scientific, 2020).

199 S. Das, Vernacular Medicine in Colonial India: Family, Market and Homoeopathy (Cambridge: Cambridge University Press, 2019).

200 S. Anderson, Making medicines: a brief history of pharmacy and pharmaceuticals (London: Pharmaceutical Press, 2005).

201 L. Monnais, The Colonial Life of Pharmaceuticals (Cambridge: Cambridge University Press, 2019).

202 Eno's Fruit Salts, John Johnson Collection of Printed Ephemera, Weston Library, Bodleian Libraries, Oxford.

203 T.A.B. Corley, 'Eno, James Crossley (1827/8–1915),' Oxford Dictionary of National Biography (2004) 2008.

204 Sanitas Advert, John Johnson Collection of Printed Ephemera, Weston Library, Bodleian Libraries, Oxford.

205 C. Hickman, 'Pine fresh: the cultural and medical context of pine scent in relation to health,' Medical Humanities 48/1 (2022), 104–13.

206 G.S. Archer, 'Enteric Carriers,' BMJ Military Health 12/3 (1909), 356.

207 W.C. Summers, Félix d'Hérelle and the origins of molecular biology (New Haven and London: Yale University Press, 1999).

208 D. Myelnikov, 'An Alternative Cure: The Adoption and Survival of Bacteriophage Therapy in the USSR, 1922–1955,' Journal of the History of Medicine and Allied Sciences 73/4 (2018), 385–411.

209 D.M. Aronoff, 'Mildred Rebstock: Profile of the Medicinal Chemist Who Synthesized Chloramphenicol,' Antimicrobial Agents and Chemotherapy 63/6 (2019), e00648-19.

210 T.E. Woodward, J.E. Smadel, H.L. Ley Jr., 'Chloramphenicol and other antibiotics in the treatment of typhoid fever and typhoid carriers,' Journal of Clinical Investigation 29/1 (1950), 87.

211 R.B. Hornick, W.E. Woodward and S.E. Greisman, 'Doctor T.E. Woodward's Legacy: From Typhus to Typhoid Fever,' Clinical Infectious Diseases 45 Suppl. 1 (2007), S6–S8.

212 H.J. Simon and R.C. Miller, 'Ampicillin in the treatment of chronic typhoid carriers: report on fifteen treated cases and a review of the literature,' NEJM 274/15 (1966), 807–15.

213 'New typhoid vaccine offers hope of protection for children,' University of Oxford (28.09.2017) [accessed: 22.12.2021].

214 A. Felix, 'Laboratory control of enteric fevers,' British Medical Bulletin 7/3 (1951), 153–62.

215 A. Felix, 'Typing of Typhoid Bacilli by Vi Bacteriophage,' BMJ 1/4292 (1943), 435.

216 C. Kirchhelle and C. Kirchhelle, 'Northern Normal – Laboratory Networks, Microbial Culture Collections, and Taxonomies of Power (1939–2000),' in A. Velmet and C. Kirchhelle eds., ESTS, forthcoming.

217 A. Hardy, 'Scientific strategy and ad hoc response: the problem of typhoid in America and England, C. 1910–50,' Journal of the history of medicine and allied sciences 69/1 (2014), 3–37.

218 W.H. Bradley, 'Epidemiological Study of Bact. typhosum Type D4,' BMJ 1/4292 (1943), 438.

219 S.H. Warren and W. Goldie, 'The Value of Vi-Phage Typing of Bact. Typhosum in investigating an outbreak of enteric fever,' EPHLS Bulletin (04.08.1945), 179–82.

220 M.J. Sikorski and M.M. Levine, 'Reviving the 'Moore Swab': A classic environmental surveillance tool involving filtration of flowing surface water and sewage water to recover typhoidal salmonella bacteria,' Applied and Environmental Microbiology 86/13 (2020), e00060-20.

221 R.P. Bernard, 'The Zermatt typhoid outbreak in 1963,' Epidemiology & Infection, 63/4 (1965), 537–63.

222 J.W. Davies et al., 'Typhoid at sea: epidemic aboard an ocean liner,' Canadian Medical Association Journal 106/8 (1972), 877.

223 P. Nicolle, 'La Lysotype de Salmonella Typhi. Son Principe, Sa Technique, Son Application À L'Épidemiologie De La Fièvre Typhoïde,' in E. Van Oye (ed.), The World Problem of Salmonellosis (Den Haag: W. Junk Publishers, 1964).

224 D.F. Smith et al., Food Poisoning, Policy and Politics. Corned Beef and Typhoid in Britain in the 1960s (Woodbridge: Boydell Press, 2005).

225 E.S. Anderson, 'The ecology of transferable drug resistance in the enterobacteria,' Annu Rev Microbiol 22 (1968), 131–80.

226 R.M. Packard, A History of Global Health: Interventions into the Lives of Other Peoples (Baltimore: Johns Hopkins University Press, 2016).

227 W. Silberstein and C.B. Gerichter, 'Salmonellosis in Israel,' in E. Van Oye (ed.), The World Problem of Salmonellosis (Den Haag: W. Junk Publishers, 1964), 335–53.

228 D. Sompolinsky et al., 'Transferable resistance factors with mutator effect in Salmonella Typhi,' Mutation Research/Fundamental and Molecular Mechanisms of Mutagenesis 4/2 (1967), 119–27.

229 K. Drlica and D.S. Perlin., Antibiotic Resistance. Understanding And Responding To An Emerging Crisis (Upper Saddle River: Pearson Education, 2011).

230 J. Colquhoun and R.S. Weetch, 'Resistance to chloramphenicol developing during treatment of typhoid fever,' Lancet 256/6639 (1950), 621–23.

231 S.H. Podolsky, The antibiotic era: reform, resistance, and the pursuit of a rational therapeutics (Baltimore: Johns Hopkins University Press, 2015).

232 C. Kirchhelle, Pyrrhic Progress: The history of antibiotics in Anglo-American food production (New Brunswick: Rutgers University Press, 2020).

233 E.S. Anderson and H.R. Smith., 'Chloramphenicol resistance in the typhoid bacillus,' BMJ 3/5822 (1972), 329–31.

234 M.C.C. Chapman, 'Comprehensive Medical Care in Vietnam,' Archives of Environmental Health: An International Journal 17/1 (1968), 21–23.

235 S.D. Airan, 'Water Supply and Wastewater Disposal In Rural Areas of India,' JAWRA 9/5 (1973), 1035–40.

236 E. Cifuentes et al., 'Epidemiologic setting of the agricultural use of sewage: Valle del Mezquital, Mexico,' *Salud publica de Mexico* 36/1 (1994), 3–9.

237 World Health Assembly, *Fifth report on the world health situation* (Geneva: WHO, 1974).

238 L.D. Willis and C. Chandler, 'Quick fix for care, productivity, hygiene and inequality: reframing the entrenched problem of antibiotic overuse,' *BMJ Global Health* 4/4 (2019), e001590.

239 OECD, *Financing water and sanitation in developing countries: the contribution of external aid* (Paris: OECD, 2010).

240 WHO, *The international drinking water supply and sanitation decade. End of decade review (as at December 1990)* (Geneva: WHO, 1992).

241 C. McMillen, '"These Findings Confirm Conclusions Many Have Arrived at by Intuition or Common Sense": Water, Quantification and Cost-effectiveness at the World Bank, c.1960 to 1995,' *Social History of Medicine* 34/2 (2021), 351–74.

242 M. Thomson, A. Kentikelenis, and T. Stubbs, 'Structural adjustment programmes adversely affect vulnerable populations: a systematic-narrative review of their effect on child and maternal health,' *Public health reviews* 38/13 (2017), 1–18.

243 M.M. Levine et al., 'Progress in vaccines against typhoid fever,' *Reviews of Infectious Diseases* 11 Suppl. 3 (1989), S552–67.

244 C.S. Waddington et al., 'Advancing the management and control of typhoid fever: a review of the historical role of human challenge studies,' *Journal of Infection* 68/5 (2014), 405–18.

245 E. Jamrozik and M.J. Selgelid, *History of Human Challenge Studies* (Springer Briefs in Ethics, 2021).

246 S.E. Greisman et al., 'Typhoid Fever: A Study of Pathogenesis and Physiologic Abnormalities,' *Transactions of the American Clinical and Climatological Association* 73 (1962), 146.

247 R. Germanier and E. Fürer, 'Isolation and Characterization of Gal E Mutant Ty 21a of Salmonella typhi: A Candidate Strain for a Live, Oral Typhoid Vaccine,' *Journal of Infectious Diseases* 131/5 (1975), 553–58.

248 R.H. Gilman et al., 'Evaluation of a UDP-glucose-4-epimeraseless mutant of Salmonella typhi as a live oral vaccine,' *Journal of Infectious Diseases* 136/6 (1977), 717–23.

249 M.M. Levine and R. Edelmann, 'Summary of an international workshop on typhoid fever,' *Reviews of Infectious Diseases* 8/3 (1986), 329–49.

250 M.M. Levine and R. Simon, 'The gathering storm: Is untreatable typhoid fever on the way?' *mBio* 9/2 (2018), e00482-18.

251 'Extensively Drug-Resistant Salmonella Typhi Infections Among U.S. Residents Without International Travel,' CDC Health Alert (12.02.2021).

252 M.J. Hughes et al. 'Extensively Drug-Resistant Typhoid Fever in the United States,' *Open Forum Infectious Diseases* 8/12 (2021), ofab572.

253 B. Rowe, L.R. Ward and E.J. Threlfall, 'Multidrug-resistant Salmonella typhi: a worldwide epidemic,' *Clinical Infectious Diseases* 24 Suppl. 1(1997), S106–09.

254 C.M. Kunin, 'Use of antimicrobial drugs in developing countries,' *International Journal of Antimicrobial Agents* 5/2 (1995), 107–13.

255 C. Kirchhelle et al., 'Setting the standard: multidisciplinary hallmarks for structural, equitable and tracked antibiotic policy,' *BMJ Global Health* 5/9 (2020), e003091.

256 S. Qureshi et al., 'Response of extensively drug resistant Salmonella Typhi to treatment with meropenem and azithromycin, in Pakistan,' *PLoS Neglected Tropical Diseases* 14/10 (2020), e0008682.

257 Data taken from salaryexplorer.com [accessed: 10.10.2021].

258 M.E. Carey et al., 'Spontaneous Emergence of Azithromycin Resistance in Independent Lineages of Salmonella Typhi in Northern India,' *Clinical Infectious Diseases* 72/5 (2021), E120–27.

259 A.C. Singer, C. Kirchhelle and A.P. Roberts, '(Inter) nationalising the antibiotic research and development pipeline,' *Lancet Infectious Diseases* 20/2 (2020), e54–e62.

260 L.R. Ochiai et al. 'The use of typhoid vaccines in Asia: the DOMI experience,' *Clinical infectious diseases* 45 Suppl. 1 (2007), S34–38.

261 D.N. Taylor et al., 'Why Are Typhoid Vaccines Not Recommended for Epidemic Typhoid Fever?' *Journal of Infectious Diseases* 180/6 (1999), 2089–90.

262 I.M. Khan et al., 'Effectiveness of Vi capsular polysaccharide typhoid vaccine among children: a cluster randomized trial in Karachi, Pakistan,' *Vaccine* 30/36 (2012), 5389–95.

263 S.A. Marathe et al., 'Typhoid fever & vaccine development: a partially answered question,' *Indian Journal of Medical Research* 135/2 (2012), 161.

264 Typhoid Immunization Working Group, *Background Paper on Vaccination against Typhoid Fever using New-Generation Vaccines – presented at the SAGE November 2007 meeting* (WHO: Geneva, 2007).

265 R. Rappuoli, E. de Gregorio and P. Costantino, 'On the mechanisms of conjugate vaccines,' *PNAS* 116/1 (2019), 14–16.

266 Z. Kossaczka et al., 'Safety and Immunogenicity of Vi Conjugate Vaccines for Typhoid Fever in Adults, Teenagers, and 2- to 4-Year-Old Children in Vietnam,' *Infection and Immunity* 67/11 (1999), 5806.

267 M.R. Capeding et al., 'Safety and immunogenicity of a Vi-DT typhoid conjugate vaccine: Phase I trial in Healthy Filipino adults and children,' *Vaccine* 36/26 (2018), 3794–3801.

268 V.K. Mohan et al., 'Safety and immunogenicity of a Vi polysaccharide-tetanus toxoid conjugate vaccine (Typbar-TCV) in healthy infants, children, and adults in typhoid endemic areas,' *Clinical Infectious Diseases* 61/3 (2015), 393–402.

269 G.J.V. Nossal, 'Vaccines of the future,' *Vaccine* 29 Suppl. 4 (2011), D111-15.

270 J.E. Meiring et al., 'Generating the Evidence for Typhoid Vaccine Introduction: Considerations for global disease burden estimates and vaccine testing through human challenge vaccine testing,' *Clinical Infectious Diseases* 69 Suppl. 5 (2019), S402–07.

271 'Millions of Children Vaccinated against Typhoid in Pakistan,' *UNICEF Pakistan* (04.3.2021) [accessed 01.04.2022].

272 M. Shakya, K.M. Neuzil and A.J. Pollard, 'Prospects of future typhoid and paratyphoid vaccines in endemic countries,' *Journal of Infectious Diseases* 224/ Suppl.7 (2021), S770–74.

273 S. Nizamuddin et al., 'Continued Outbreak of Ceftriaxone-Resistant Salmonella enterica Serotype Typhi across Pakistan and Assessment of Knowledge and Practices among Healthcare Workers,' *American Journal of Tropical Medicine and Hygiene* 104/4 (2021), 1265–70.

ACKNOWLEDGEMENTS

THIS BOOK is the fruit of five years of learning and collaboration across disciplinary and international borders. Together with my co-curator, Samantha Vanderslott, I am grateful to the Oxford Martin School, Oxford Vaccine Group, University College Dublin's School of History and the New Venture Fund for enabling us to turn a small interdisciplinary workshop into a large international research and engagement project. It has been an honour to work on the Typhoidland exhibitions with partners across three continents. We owe particular thanks to the University of Oxford's History of Science Museum and Weston Library, the Museum of Oxford, the David J. Sencer CDC Museum, St John's Research Institute in Bengaluru, Patan Hospital in Nepal and the Child Health Research Foundation in Dhaka. This book is rooted in the stimulating collaborative research underpinning our Typhoidland exhibitions. Working with Sam and learning from colleagues across many institutions has been hugely enjoyable. I am particularly grateful to Emily Webster, Kate Emary, Arabella Stuart, Sam Martin, Sean Elias, Margaret Pelling, Christoph Gradmann, Andrew Pollard and François-Xavier Weill, whose valuable insights helped transform a very rough draft into a readable manuscript. All remaining mistakes are my own. Finally, my family has been a rock of endless support during the many academic and personal stages of the Typhoidland journey. Since starting out on the project in October 2017, two children have been born, a pandemic has swept the world and we have moved countries and jobs. Charlotte was never too tired to read through texts, tweak figures or take over childcare, while Clara and Emil were a source of endless joy – and distraction. I hope that readers will not only enjoy this book as much as I enjoyed writing it, but also come away with an appreciation of the ongoing challenge posed by typhoid and the potential of collective action to shorten its future.

Image credits

p.4: George Eliot Archive; **p.6**: CDC Image Library; **p.8**: Wellcome Collection; **p.9**: CDC Image Library; **p.10**: Adapted from Ohad Gal-Mor, *Clinical Microbiology Reviews*, 2019; **p.11**: Wellcome Collection; **p.12**: Wellcome Collection; **p.14**: Wellcome Collection; **p.16**: Portrait from Fielding Hudson Garrison, *An introduction to the history of medicine* (London & Philadelphia: W.B. Saunders, 1914); **p.18**: Wellcome Collection; **p.20**: John Johnson Collection, Public Services Box No. 5, Weston Library, University of Oxford; **p.22**: Wellcome Collection; **p.23**: Snow, J. *On the Mode of Communication of Cholera*, 2nd Edition, 1855; **p.24**: Wikicommons; **p.27**: Wellcome Collection; **p.28**: Curschmann, H., Osler, W., Stengel, A., *Typhoid fever and typhus fever* (Philadelphia and London: W.B. Saunders and Company, 1901); **p.30**: CDC Image Library; **p.31**: Typhoidland Collection; **p.32**: Wellcome Collection; **p.34**: History of Science Museum, Oxford; **p.36 (top)**: Print of the Oxford Almanack 1894, Oxford University Images; **p.36 (bottom)**: Oxfordshire History Centre, ref: D267117a; **p.37 (top)**: © British Library Board. All Rights Reserved / Bridgeman Images; **p.37 (bottom)**: L. Carroll, *Through the Looking-Glass, and What Alice Found There* (London: Macmillan, 1871); **p.40**: Oxford City Council, OCA3/1/Y1/41/6 (above); Oxford City Council, OCA3/1/Y1/41/5 (below); **p.41**: Digital composite by Claas Kirchhelle and Mike Athanson of original maps from the Bodleian Libraries and the Oxford City Council Archives (Typhoidland collection); **p.43**: Historic England, EAW003957; **p.44**: Oxfordshire History Centre; **p.45**: Digital composite by Claas Kirchhelle and Michael Athanson based on Oxford's Medical Office of Health Annual Reports and census data held at the Oxfordshire History Centre (Typhoidland Collection); **p.46**: CDC Image Library; **p.48 (top)**: George Whipple and William Thompson Sedgwick, *Typhoid Fever: Its Causation, Transmission and Prevention* (New York: Wiley & Sons, 1908), 9; **p.48 (bottom)**: Harpenden and District Local History Society; **p.49**: National Library of Ireland, CLAR116; **p.50**: 'Where Grim Death Daily Lurks', in Cory, J. Campbell, 'The Cartoonist's Art, in Which the First and Last Word Is Spoken,' (Chicago: Tumbo Co., 1912) Print, 40; **p.51**: Wellcome Collection; **p.53**: *New York American*, 29 June 1909; **p.55**: Science History Images/Alamy; **p.56 (top)**: New York State Archives, Aerial photographic prints and negatives of New York State sites, 1941–57, B1598–99. Box 8, no. 52; **p.56 (bottom x2)**: NYC Department of Records & Information Services; **p.58**: W. McLean and E.H. Shackleton, *O.H.M.S., or How 1200 Soldiers went to Table Bay* (London: Simpkin, Marshall, Hamilton, Kent & Company, 1900); **p.60**: Wikicommons; **p.62**: Wellcome Collection; **p.63**: Images from the History of Medicine (NLM Digital Collections); **p.64**: Imperial War Museum Q114677; **p.65**: 'Herstellung des Typhusimpfstoffs', *Die Woche* (13.02.1915), 247–48; **p.67**: John Johnson Collection, Weston Library, University of Oxford; **pp.68–71, 72 (top)**: John Johnson Collection of Printed Ephemera, Bodleian Library; **p.72 (bottom)**: Wikicommons; **p.73**: Wellcome Collection; **p.74**: Gates Archive/Samantha Reinders; **p.76**: Science Museum. 1996-402; **p.77**: John Oxley Library, State Library of Queensland; **p.78 (top)**: CDC Image Library; **p.78 (bottom)**: Images from the History of Medicine (NLM Digital Collections); **pp.80, 81, 83**: Wellcome Collection; **p.86**: University of Oxford, photo: Andrew Testa; **pp.87, 89**: Gates Archive/Samantha Reinders; **p.90**: Coalition Against Typhoid, 2021.

The quotes on p.69 are from the John Johnson Collection of Printed Ephemera, Bodleian Library.